Barbara Bruce, Ph.D.
W. Michael Hooten, M.D.

Medical Editors-in-Chief

Mayo Clinic
Rochester, Minnesota

Published by Mayo Clinic Health Solutions

© 2008 Mayo Foundation for Medical Education and Research

For bulk sales to employers, member groups and health-related companies, contact Mayo Clinic Health Management Resources, 200 First St. S.W., Rochester, MN, 55905, or send an e-mail to SpecialSalesMayoBooks@Mayo.edu.

Address inquiries to Mayo Clinic Health Solutions, Permissions Department, 200 First St. S.W., Fifth Floor Centerplace Building, Rochester, MN, 55905.

Stock photography from Artville, BananaStock, Brand X Pictures, Comstock, Corbis, Creatas, Digital Stock, Digital Vision, Eyewire, Food Shapes, Image Ideas, © Isabelle Rozenbaum/PhotoAlto, Photodisc, Rubberball and Stockbyte. The individuals pictured are models, and the photos are used for illustrative purposes only. There's no correlation between the individuals portrayed and the subjects being discussed.

Library of Congress Control Number: 2007937326

Printed in Canada

First Edition

3 4 5 6 7 8 9 10

About Mayo Clinic

Mayo Clinic evolved from the frontier practice of Dr. William Worrall Mayo and the partnership of his two sons, Drs. William J. and Charles H. Mayo, in the early 1900s. Pressed by the demands of their busy practice in Rochester, Minn., the Mayo brothers invited other physicians to join them, pioneering the private group practice of medicine. Today, with more than 2,000 physicians and scientists at three major locations in Rochester, Minn., Jacksonville, Fla., and Scottsdale, Ariz., Mayo Clinic is dedicated to providing comprehensive diagnoses, accurate answers and effective treatments.

With this depth of medical knowledge, experience and expertise, Mayo Clinic occupies an unparalleled position as a health information resource. Since 1983, Mayo Clinic has published reliable health information for millions of consumers through a variety of award-winning newsletters, books and online services. Revenue from these publishing activities supports Mayo Clinic programs, including medical education and medical research.

Editorial staff

Preface

Accurate and useful information is vital to maintaining good health and managing illness. This is particularly true for the common and often-complicated problem of chronic pain.

Advances in the field of pain medicine are occurring rapidly. *Mayo Clinic Guide to Pain Relief* includes information on how the nervous system responds to painful illness and injury and describes common pain conditions such as low back pain, migraines and fibromyalgia. This book emphasizes a take-charge approach to managing persistent pain by providing detailed information and instructions on exercise, daily activities, behavior therapies and stress reduction techniques. Complementary and alternative medicine approaches for coping with chronic pain also are reviewed.

The pain management strategies presented in this book are based on the expertise of Mayo Clinic physicians, psychologists, nurses, and physical and occupational therapists. We are indebted to the staff of Mayo Clinic's Pain Rehabilitation Center, Pain Clinic and Fibromyalgia Treatment Program for their guidance and assistance.

We believe you'll find this book to be a helpful and practical resource for effectively managing your pain. Your knowledge and use of pain management strategies, together with the support of family and friends and the guidance of your personal physician, offer you the best opportunity for enjoying the pain relief you seek.

Barbara Bruce, Ph.D.
Medical editor-in-chief

W. Michael Hooten, M.D.
Medical editor-in-chief

Table of contents

Part 1   Understanding chronic pain 11

Chapter 1   About this book 13
How to use this book 15
The three parts 16

Chapter 2   What is pain? 19
How you feel pain 21
Your pain response 24
Acute pain vs. chronic pain 27
What causes chronic pain? 28
Sensitization 29
Chronic pain challenges 30

Chapter 3   Common types of chronic pain 31
Arthritis 31
Back pain 34
Complex regional pain syndrome 36
Fibromyalgia 37
Headache 37
Irritable bowel syndrome 40
Mouth, jaw and face pain 41
Neck pain 43
Overuse strain injuries 44
Peripheral neuropathy 48
Postherpetic neuralgia 49
Unknown causes 49

Chapter 4   **Chronic pain cycles** **51**

Behavioral cycle 52

Emotional cycle 55

Your family's responses 58

Breaking the cycles 60

Chapter 5   **Costs of chronic pain** **61**

Physical deconditioning 62

Loss of sleep 62

Emotional upheaval 63

Depression 64

Difficulties at work 65

Financial strain 66

Damaged relationships 66

Substance misuse 67

Taking one step at a time 68

Part 2   **Treating chronic pain** **69**

Chapter 6   **Medication** **71**

About pain medications 72

Wise use of medications 74

Simple pain relievers 76

Opioids (narcotics) 79

Topical medications 84

Other pain medications 86

Emotional symptoms 90

Related physical conditions 93

The benefits vs. the risks 94

Chapter 7   **Injections, stimulators and pumps** **95**

Injection therapy 95

Nerve stimulators 105

Medication pumps 108

Choosing the right treatment 109

Chapter 8 **Pain specialists** **111**

What's a pain specialist? 112

What's a pain clinic? 113

Working as a team 114

What to look for 115

Chapter 9 **Pain rehabilitation centers** **117**

Rehabilitation programs 117

What to expect 119

Chapter 10 **Complementary and alternative medicine** **123**

5 smart strategies 124

Herbs and other supplements 126

Hands-on therapies 129

Energy therapies 133

Mind-body therapies 135

Part 3

Managing chronic pain **141**

Chapter 11 **Developing a pain control program** **143**

Start with SMART goals 144

Put it in writing 146

Going forward 149

Chapter 12 **Staying active with daily exercise** **151**

Flexibility exercises 153

Stretching exercises 154

Strengthening exercises 158

How to make it work 163

Chapter 13   **Finding balance: Planning and moderation 167**

How does your day balance out? 169
Put time on your side 169
Get more organized 173
Do everything in moderation 173
Develop better daily habits 174
Move your body wisely 177

Chapter 14   **Dealing with your emotions and behaviors 181**

Admitting your loss 182
Dealing with depression 183
Managing your anxiety 187
Managing your anger 188
Challenging your expectations 190
Learning to assert yourself 190
Boosting your self-esteem 193
Responding to your behaviors 194
Responding to your emotions 194

Chapter 15   **Managing stress 197**

What stress does to you 198
What are your stress triggers? 198
How to stress less 200
Learn how to relax 202

Chapter 16   **Interacting with family and friends 205**

Building bridges 206
Talking openly and honestly 207
How family and friends can help you 209

Chapter 17   **Caring for yourself 211**

Getting a good night's sleep 211
Controlling your weight 216
Eating better 221

Limiting alcohol 223
Quitting smoking 224
Expressing your sexuality 228
Addressing your spiritual needs 231

Chapter 18 Staying in control **233**
Getting through bad days 234
10 ways to maintain your gains 235

Additional resources **239**
Glossary **243**
Index **249**

Understanding chronic pain

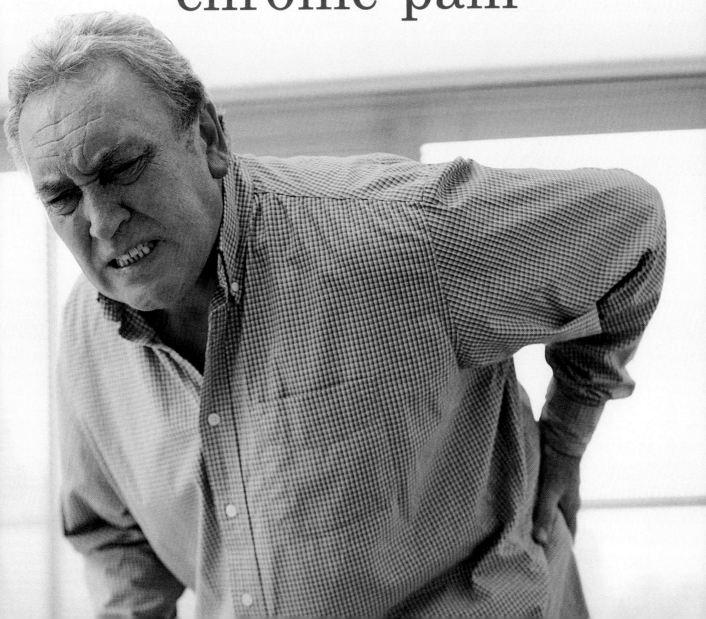

Chapter 1

About this book

When you're in pain, there's nothing you want more than relief from the constant throbbing, stinging or aching. With many types of injuries and illnesses, given time, the pain will eventually disappear. But not all pain can be eliminated. For some people, the pain never goes away. Does this mean you can never experience pain relief? No, it doesn't. But it does mean you may have to change your definition of *relief*.

With some types of chronic, or persistent, pain, medications and interventions are available that can produce a major reduction in pain, and possibly even get rid of the pain altogether. In other instances, however, nothing seems to work. No matter what the

treatment — pills, a shot, surgery — the pain endures. But even in this situation, you can still experience pain relief. Given the right tools and techniques, you can reduce the aching and throbbing to a more tolerable level — one that you can live with.

Mayo Clinic Guide to Pain Relief is a comprehensive, how-to pain control manual. Whether you've lived with chronic pain for years or have recently been diagnosed, this book can supply you with the information and tools you need to eliminate or lessen your pain. Our hope is that this book will make you a better consumer of medical care for your pain, regardless of the type of pain you're experiencing or how long you've been searching for pain relief.

While the focus of this book is on the treatment of chronic pain, we also provide up-to-date information on treatments used to treat short-term (acute) pain that follows surgery or an accident, such as a broken bone.

Why is managing pain important? Pain can interfere with your enjoyment of life. It can make it difficult to sleep, work, socialize with friends and family and accomplish everyday tasks. When your ability to function is limited, you may become less productive. Ongoing pain can cause you to lose your appetite, feel weak and depressed. You may also find yourself avoiding hobbies and other enjoyable activities in order to prevent further injury or pain. But while your pain may be part of you, it doesn't have to destroy you.

By learning how to manage your pain, you can reclaim your life and become some or all of the person that you used to be. This book is about helping you find the relief you seek.

How to use this book

Mayo Clinic Guide to Pain Relief emphasizes a take-charge approach to successfully managing chronic pain by providing detailed information and instructions on a variety of strategies for controlling pain. These include daily exercise, activity modification, stress reduction techniques, behavior changes and goal setting. The book also discusses when medications may be useful and why many times medications aren't the answer to long-term pain control.

Your level of pain and how much it's affecting your ability to function will determine how best to use this book. If you've just begun to experience persistent pain, you may find the discussion of how pain develops and various treatments for chronic pain most helpful. If you've been battling chronic pain for years and have concluded that medications don't help or they cause unwanted side effects, the last section of the book on pain management strategies can teach you how to better manage your pain without medication.

However, regardless of your pain type or its severity, the best way to use this book and to gain the most from it, is to read it from beginning to end — and return to it as needed.

The three parts

Mayo Clinic Guide to Pain Relief is divided into three sections, or parts. The first section provides valuable background to help you better understand why you're in pain. The second section focuses on medical treatments and therapies that can help control pain. The third section is the "what you can do" portion of the book. This section addresses specific steps you can take to help relieve your pain.

Part 1: Understanding chronic pain

To control your pain, you need to understand how pain develops, what influences pain and why some pain persists. Part 1 discusses the anatomy of pain — the parts of your body involved in the development of pain — and why some people respond to pain differently than do others. There's also information on conditions and illnesses commonly associated with chronic pain, as well as a discussion of the long-term physical, emotional and financial effects of ongoing pain.

Part 2: Treating chronic pain

There are many options for treating pain. The most common is medication. Part 2 begins with a discussion of various drugs used to relieve pain. You can learn why some medications are generally more effective for certain types of pain than are others. You'll also read about the potential side effects of some pain medications, especially if the drugs are taken in large doses or over the long term.

In addition, Part 2 reviews other types of treatments used to relieve pain, such as injections given at pain sites, nerve stimulators and medication pumps, as well as alternative and complementary therapies. If you're considering seeing a pain specialist or your primary care doctor has recommended that you do so, there's a discussion of the different types of pain clinics, centers and programs available and what to look for to find the right one for you.

Part 3: Managing chronic pain

With chronic pain, there often isn't an effective treatment for the pain — a medication or some other form of therapy that can make the pain disappear. The next step then becomes learning how to live with the pain.

Part 3 focuses on steps you can take to manage your pain so that it doesn't interfere with your ability to work, spend time with family and friends, or enjoy life. And what people have found is that when their pain is no longer the focus of their attention, its severity tends to decrease. Some of the strategies for managing chronic pain discussed in Part 3 include goal setting, daily exercise, activity modification, emotional and behavioral changes, positive thinking, stress management, sleep improvement, healthy eating, weight control and improved family relationships.

Consider Part 3 the self-help section of the book. This is where you'll find information on steps that you can take on your own to get yourself on course to life with less pain.

Chapter 2

What is pain?

Pain is a universal experience. We all feel it, whether it's the sharp, stabbing pain of a twisted ankle or the deep, throbbing pain of a headache that won't quit. Pain knows no age limit — it affects us from infancy through old age. More than one in four Americans reports experiencing at least one episode of persistent pain that lasts more than 24 hours.

What exactly is pain? Pain is defined as "an unpleasant sensory and emotional experience associated with actual or potential tissue damage, or described in terms of such damage." Sensitivity to pain is complex and varies from person to person. An experience that may cause one person immediate, excruciating pain may result in only minor discomfort for another. This varied sensitivity can sometimes make pain hard to describe. The degree to which you feel pain and how you react to it are the results of your biological, psychological and cultural makeup. In addition, past encounters with a painful injury or illness can influence your sensitivity to pain.

There are times when pain can be useful — almost protective — such as when it warns you that the hot skillet you've just picked up will burn your hand if you don't put it down quickly. But other pain — the day-after-day chronic ache of arthritis or the constant throbbing of a headache — seems to serve no useful purpose. And its relentlessness can be overwhelming.

When pain persists beyond the time expected for an injury to heal or an illness to end, it can become a chronic condition. No longer is the pain viewed as the symptom of another disease, rather it's seen as an illness unto itself. This type of pain is known as chronic pain, or chronic noncancer pain in order to distinguish it from cancer (malignant) pain. Other names include chronic pain syndrome or chronic benign pain, though nothing about it may seem benign.

Chronic pain can be difficult to treat. Often, medication alone isn't sufficient to help people struggling with chronic pain. In most instances, a comprehensive approach is used, which may include medication, physical therapy,

Making sense of your nervous system

Your nervous system is composed of nerve cells and fibers that transmit and receive messages in the form of electrical currents and chemical interactions. It's through this intricate web of cells that your body and brain communicate.

Two main components make up your nervous system: your central nervous system, which includes your brain and spinal cord, and your peripheral nervous system. Your peripheral nerves extend from your spinal cord to your skin, muscles and internal organs. Within each of these systems are three major categories of nerves:

- **Autonomic nerves** maintain normal body processes, such as breathing, heart rate, blood pressure, digestion, perspiration and sexual function.
- **Motor nerves** are responsible for movement of your muscles. They allow you to move your hands and feet, to walk or to sit.
- **Sensory nerves** are your sensing nerves. They allow you to feel an object when you touch it. They're also the nerves that allow you to feel pain.

psychological and behavioral therapy, and interventional treatments such as injections and nerve blocks.

The good news, though, is that despite having persistent pain, you can still enjoy an active, productive and satisfying lifestyle.

Managing chronic pain has evolved from a time when it was thought that pain was something to be tolerated and endured, and that complaining or seeking relief was a sign of weakness. Medical practice has determined that pain is something that should be considered when evaluating the basic condition of a person seeking medical care. In fact, pain has been termed the *fifth vital sign* and doctors are urged to assess their patients for pain at the same time they check a patient's four main vital signs — pulse, blood pressure, body temperature and respiration.

The U.S. Congress has declared the current decade the Decade of Pain Control and Research. The Joint Commission — formerly known as the Joint Commission on Accreditation of Healthcare Organizations (JCAHO) — which sets and enforces standards of care in hospitals and other health care facilities, has a list of 10 standards designed to ensure the assessment and treatment of pain for every patient.

This book can help you better understand your pain and its harmful effects, and perhaps more importantly, it explains how you can take control of your pain — instead of letting it control you.

How you feel pain

Understanding the mechanism that causes your body to produce pain can help you better appreciate why it is that you experience pain. It can also help you better understand why chronic pain is often difficult to treat.

Pain basically results from a series of electrical and chemical exchanges involving three major components: your peripheral nerves, spinal cord and brain.

Peripheral nerves

Your peripheral (pe-RIF-er-ul) nerves encompass a network of nerve fibers that branches throughout your body. Attached to some of these fibers are special nerve endings that can sense an unpleasant stimulus, such as a cut, burn or painful pressure. These nerve endings are called nociceptors (no-sih-SEP-turs).

You have millions of nociceptors in your skin, bones, joints and muscles and in the protective membrane around your internal organs. Nociceptors are concentrated in areas more prone to injury, such as your fingers and toes. That's why a splinter in your finger hurts more than one in your back or shoulder. There may be as many as

1,300 nociceptors in just one square inch of skin. Muscles, protected beneath your skin, have fewer nerve endings. And internal organs, protected by skin, muscle and bone, have fewer still.

Some nociceptors sense sharp blows, others heat. One type senses pressure, temperature and chemical changes. Nociceptors can also detect inflammation caused by injury, disease or infection.

When nociceptors detect a harmful stimulus, they relay their pain messages

2. Pain messages move through peripheral nerves and up the spinal cord.

3. Your brain interprets the messages as pain, including its location, intensity and nature (burning, aching, stinging).

4. Your brain sends pain-suppressing chemicals to the pain source and triggers other responses.

1. Pain source.

The pain pathway

Pain results from a series of electrical and chemical changes involving your peripheral nerves, spinal cord and brain.

in the form of electrical impulses along a peripheral nerve to your spinal cord and brain. However, the speed by which the messages travel can vary. Sensations of severe pain are transmitted almost instantaneously. Dull, aching pain — such as an upset stomach or an earache — is relayed on fibers that transmit at a slower speed.

Spinal cord

When pain messages reach your spinal cord, they meet up with specialized nerve cells that act as gatekeepers. The nerve cells filter the pain messages on their way to your brain.

For severe pain that's linked to bodily harm, such as when you touch a hot stove, the "gate" is wide open and the messages take an express route to your brain. Nerve cells in your spinal cord also respond to these urgent warnings by triggering other parts of the nervous system into action, such as your motor nerves. Your motor nerves signal your muscles to pull your hand away from the burner. Weak pain messages, however, such as from a scratch, may be filtered or blocked out by the gate.

Within your spinal cord, the messages can also change. Other sensations may

overpower and diminish the pain signals, such as when you massage the injured area. The warnings sent by your peripheral nerves are downgraded to a lower priority. Nerve cells in your spinal cord may also release chemicals that amplify or diminish the messages, affecting the strength of the pain signal.

Brain

When pain messages reach your brain, they arrive at the thalamus, a sorting and switching station deep inside your brain. The thalamus interprets the messages as pain and forwards them simultaneously to three specialized regions: the physical sensation region (somatosensory cortex), the emotional and feeling region (limbic system) and the thinking region (frontal cortex). Your awareness of pain becomes a complex experience affected by these three regions.

Your brain responds to the pain messages by sending back messages that promote the healing process. For instance, if you've cut your finger, your brain signals your autonomic nervous system, the system that controls blood flow, to send additional blood and nutrients to the injury site.

It also dispatches the release of pain-suppressing chemicals and sends stop-pain messages to the injury site.

Your pain response

When pain messages reach your brain, two things generally determine how you respond to them — the physical sensation associated with the messages and your individual characteristics.

Physical sensation

Pain results when pain receptors in your body become injured or inflamed due to an injury or illness. Pain comes in many forms: sharp, jabbing, throbbing, burning, stinging, tingling, nagging, dull and aching. It also varies from mild to severe. Severe pain grabs your attention quickly and often produces a greater physical and emotional response than does mild pain. Severe pain can also incapacitate you, making it difficult or impossible to sit or stand.

However, physical sensation associated with pain is more than just the effects

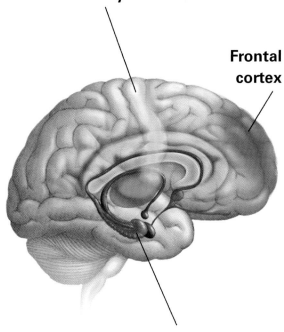

Somatosensory cortex

Frontal cortex

Limbic system

Your brain and pain

Three areas of your brain influence how you respond to pain. The somatosensory cortex deciphers the physical sensation — is the pain sharp and jabbing or dull and aching? The limbic system controls your emotional response to pain — do you cry out in agony or disregard it as a minor annoyance? The frontal cortex is responsible for your physical reaction, such as pulling your hand away from a hot burner or rubbing a bump on your head.

of tissue damage. Pain pathways that travel through your spinal cord also pass through a number of areas within your brain, affecting how you experience pain. As pain messages travel through the brain's emotional and feeling region (limbic system) and thinking region (frontal cortex) they may be altered by a number of factors such as anxiety, fear, past pain experiences and the pain experiences of loved ones.

Individuality

People respond to pain in different ways because pain is made up of many unique components. Equally important in the experience of pain is who you are. Your reaction to pain is heavily influenced by your personal traits and characteristics.

An injury or illness that may be very painful for one person may only be

Natural painkillers and pain enhancers

Your brain and spinal cord produce their own painkillers, which are similar to the narcotic drug morphine, used to treat severe pain. Two types of morphine-like pain relievers are endorphins (en-DOR-fins) and enkephalins (en-KEF-uh-lins). When released, these substances attach to special receptors in your brain, producing stop-pain messages.

Other substances in your body do the opposite. They intensify your pain. A protein called substance P stimulates nerve endings at the injury site and within your spinal cord, increasing pain messages. Other pain enhancers work by activating normally silent nerve cells in the injured area. This activation prompts the cells to discharge pain messages even when the stimulation they detect isn't painful. This not only worsens the pain but also enlarges the area of sensitivity.

slightly bothersome for another. Why is this? Many factors are believed to affect how you sense and react to pain. Your personal genetics, including how sensitive your body is to pain signals is a key component. Other factors include how you think, learn and reason; your expectations as to how you "think" you should feel; how attentive you are to your body's responses — what your body seems to be telling you; and whether you're dealing with other illnesses or conditions, such as depression or anxiety, that can affect how you sense and react to pain.

In addition, memories of past painful experiences, cultural factors, and your upbringing and attitude also affect how you interpret pain messages and tolerate pain. For example, a minor sensation that would barely register as pain, such as a dentist's probe, can actually produce exaggerated pain for a child who's never been to the dentist and is nervous about it.

But your emotional state can also work in your favor, improving even a severe pain experience. This was illustrated by a study that compared formerly wounded war veterans with men in the general population. Men in both groups had the same kind of surgery.

The combat veterans, however, required less pain medication than the others did, perhaps because they thought that the surgery was a minor matter compared with what they'd experienced in battle.

So, pain literally is "in your head." There's no way to disentangle tissue damage due to injury or illness from the complex emotional and cognitive processing that accompanies the pain experience.

Acute pain vs. chronic pain

There are two major categories of pain. Acute pain is triggered by tissue damage and is designed to protect you from further injury. Acute pain is the type of pain that generally accompanies illness, injury or surgery. It may be mild and last just a moment, such as from a sting. Or it can be severe and last for weeks or months, such as from a burn, pulled muscle or broken bone.

With acute pain, you typically know exactly where it hurts — the term *acute* refers to a sharp pain. A toothache

from a cavity, a burning elbow from a scrape and pain from a surgical incision are examples of acute pain. With time and treatment of the underlying cause, the pain generally fades away — when the cavity is filled, the skin grows back or the incision heals.

Chronic pain refers to persistent pain — pain that continues after the injury is healed. Pain is generally described as chronic when it lasts six months or longer. This is reflected in the word itself. Chronic comes from the Greek word for "time."

As with acute pain, chronic pain spans the full range of sensations and intensity. It can feel tingling, jolting, burning, dull or sharp. The pain may remain constant or come and go, like a migraine that develops without warning.

Unlike acute pain, however, with chronic pain you may not know the reason for the pain. The original injury shows every indication of being healed, yet the pain remains — and may be even more intense.

Chronic pain can also occur without any indication of injury. Years ago, people who complained of pain that had no apparent cause were thought to be imagining the misery or trying to get attention. Doctors now know that's not true. Chronic pain is real.

What causes chronic pain?

Frequently, the cause of chronic pain isn't well understood. There may be no evidence of disease or damage to your body tissues that doctors can directly link to the pain.

Sometimes, chronic pain is due to a chronic condition, such as arthritis, which produces painful inflammation in your joints, fibromyalgia, which causes aching in your muscles, or a migraine, which causes swelling of blood vessels in your brain and scalp.

Occasionally, chronic pain may stem from an accident, infection or surgery that damages a peripheral or spinal nerve. This type of nerve pain that lingers after the original injury heals is called neuropathic — meaning the damaged nerve, not the original injury, is causing the pain. Neuropathic pain can also result from diseases such as diabetes or alcoholism.

Once damaged, the nerve may send pain messages that are unwarranted. For example, metabolic changes associated with diabetes can damage the small nerves in your hands and feet, producing a tingling and painful burning sensation.

Little is known about why injured nerves sometimes misfire and send painful messages. However, one reason is that when a nerve is destroyed, the severed end can sprout a tangle of unorganized nerve fibers (neuroma). This bundle of nerve tissue then starts sending spontaneous pain signals. These fibers also refuse to follow normal checks and balances that keep pain at bay.

Sensitization

Scientific research continues to provide new knowledge of how pain is transmitted and how the experience of pain is created in the brain.

One important aspect of these new discoveries about pain has to do with a process called sensitization. An introduction to sensitization can help you to understand why it is that chronic pain

can be so severe and why your pain may seem out of proportion to the type of injury or disease that you experienced.

The intricate biology involved in sensitization is complex, but the basic idea behind it is fairly straightforward. When pain signals are transmitted from injured or diseased tissues to the brain, during transmission these signals may activate (sensitize) pain circuits in other locations such as the peripheral nerves and spinal cord.

The process of sensitization can be compared to the volume control on your stereo, amplifying — and sometimes distorting — the pain message. The result is a painful condition that's severe and out of proportion to the disease or original injury. Sensitization may affect all regions of your nervous system that process pain messages, including the sensing, feeling and thinking centers of the brain. When this occurs, chronic pain also may be associated with emotional and psychological suffering.

An example of sensitization is phantom limb pain. In this condition, a person can feel intense pain in the location of a missing body part, for example, an arm or a leg that has been amputated. The difficult-to-treat problem of phantom limb pain is explained by persistent activation (sensitization) in the pain transmission pathways anywhere from the site of amputation to the brain.

Considerable scientific research around the world is focused on identifying the molecular and cellular processes that cause sensitization. The results of this research are likely to provide new and better treatments for many types of chronic pain.

Chronic pain challenges

Because pain is such a personal experience, persistent pain can be difficult to treat. Occasionally, surgery can cure or reduce pain. And for some types of chronic pain, medication or injections are beneficial. Frequently, though, none of these approaches are very effective.

But that doesn't mean there isn't any hope. Treatments may not make your pain disappear, but you can learn how to manage your pain and improve your quality of life.

Living well despite chronic pain has a lot to do with your attitude and lifestyle. If you have a negative attitude and view yourself as a victim of your pain, the pain will continue to control you and consume your energy. On the other hand, if you approach your condition with a positive attitude and a willingness to change, you're likely to be successful in coping with your pain.

In the chapters that follow, we provide key steps to help you live better with chronic pain. Not only can this book help you discover what may be contributing to your pain, it also includes strategies and suggestions for how to make positive life changes. With your doctor, other health care professionals, and your family and friends, you can learn to take control of your pain — and your life.

Chapter 3

Common types of chronic pain

Chronic pain can affect just about any part of your body, from your head to your toes, from your skin to your internal organs. Your pain may be related to an existing illness or stem from an accident or injury. Perhaps your pain is linked to a condition that doctors don't fully understand. Or maybe it has no apparent cause.

Arthritis pain, back pain and headache are the most common types of chronic pain, but many other conditions can produce persistent pain. In this chapter, we discuss some of the more common disorders and diseases that can lead to chronic pain and what may be the culprit behind the pain.

Arthritis

The term *arthritis* means "joint inflammation." Although people often talk about it as one disease, it's not. There are many forms of arthritis. Some forms begin gradually. Others appear suddenly and then disappear, only to return again later.

Arthritis can affect any joint in your body and it may be triggered by various causes, including an injury, lack of physical activity, natural wear on your joints or genetic disease. The two most common forms of arthritis are osteoarthritis and rheumatoid arthritis.

Osteoarthritis

About half of all people with arthritis have osteoarthritis, which affects approximately 21 million Americans. This condition results when cartilage that cushions the ends of bones in your joints deteriorates. If the cartilage wears down completely, you may be left with bone rubbing against bone, irritating the joint and producing pain.

Your body tries to repair the damage, but often the repairs are unsuccessful, resulting in growth of new bone along the sides of existing bone. The new bone may produce bony lumps, most noticeably in your hands and feet, and especially in the joints of your fingers and toes. These lumps, called spurs, may or may not produce pain and tenderness.

Osteoarthritis most often develops after age 45 and occurs equally in men and women. It can develop anywhere in your body, but it tends to be most common in your hands and feet, neck, lower back, knees and hips. The disease generally is associated with wear

Normal spine

- Disk
- Nerve
- Vertebra

Spine with osteoarthritis

- Bone spur
- Narrowed disk

Osteoarthritis

Elastic structures called disks serve as cushions between vertebrae in a normal spine, keeping it flexible. In osteoarthritis, disks narrow, leading to bony lumps along the edges of vertebrae, called spurs. Pain and stiffness may occur where bone surfaces rub together.

on your joints or a specific injury to a joint. It may also stem from an imbalance of enzymes in a joint, causing cartilage to break down.

Initially, arthritis pain may be minor and hurt only when you use the affected joint. In time, the pain can intensify and hurt even when you're not using the joint.

Rheumatoid arthritis

Unlike osteoarthritis, rheumatoid arthritis is thought to stem from an immune system disorder that causes your immune system to attack the lining in your joints.

White blood cells move into joint tissues, producing inflammation and pain. Swelling of the tissues triggers the release of natural chemicals that can damage cartilage, tendons and ligaments. Gradually, the joint loses its shape. In some cases, the disease destroys the joint.

Rheumatoid arthritis most often affects joints in your wrists, hands, feet and

Thickened synovial membrane

Synovial fluid

Degraded cartilage

Rheumatoid arthritis

Rheumatoid arthritis often leads to deformity of the fingers and hands. During flare-ups of the disease, your hands may be painful and weak.

ankles. It can also affect your elbows, shoulders, hips, knees, neck and jaw. In addition to pain and swelling, you may experience stiffness and loss of motion in the joints.

The disease typically develops between ages 20 and 50. An estimated 2 million Americans have rheumatoid arthritis, and roughly twice as many women as men are affected by it.

Back pain

Four out of five adults have at least one bout of back pain during their lifetime. And millions of Americans experience back pain on a frequent basis. In fact, back pain is one of the most common reasons for health care visits and missed work.

Most back pain occurs in your lower back (lumbar area), which bears most of your weight. Your lower back also serves as your body's pivot point, allowing you to bend forward and backward and twist sideways.

Acute back pain often stems from an injury or overuse. Usually, there's an accumulation of stress with one partic-

ular event causing the pain. Sometimes, though, back pain can occur for no specific reason and frequently recur. This is often referred to as chronic non-specific back pain. What causes some people to experience this type of pain isn't always clear. Oftentimes, back pain is related to one of the following conditions.

Muscle strain and spasm

Muscle strain is a common cause of back pain — especially pain in the lower back. Muscle strain can occur if you lift something too heavy, twist too sharply or stand on your feet too long. Excess body weight and poor posture also can lead to muscle strain. When your back muscles become strained, they also can spasm, or "knot up." Spasm is your back's response to injury, designed to immobilize you and prevent further damage. Any movement of the injured muscles can set off a wave of stabbing pains.

The good news is that approximately 90 percent of these strains resolve within four weeks, usually much sooner. The remaining 10 percent take longer to heal. In some cases, the pain never goes away and becomes a chronic problem.

Sciatica

This condition is named for the sciatic (si-AT-ic) nerve that extends down each leg from your buttock to your heel. Inflammation or compression of a nerve root in your lower back can cause sciatica. You may feel the pain radiating from your back down through your buttock to your lower leg. Tingling, numbness or muscle weakness also may occur. Another cause of sciatica is related to spasms or tightness in the buttock (gluteal) muscles. This is called piriformis syndrome.

Usually, the pain goes away on its own. However, severe nerve compression can cause progressive muscle weakness and continued pain.

Herniated disk

Injury or normal wear and tear can cause a disk between the bones in your back (vertebrae) to bulge or rupture. This is sometimes called a slipped disk.

Sciatic nerve

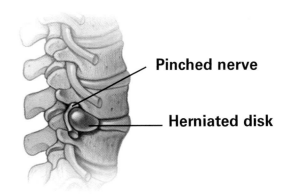

Pinched nerve

Herniated disk

Sciatica

Sciatica is pain that radiates from your back down through your buttock to your lower leg. It may be caused by inflammation or compression of spinal nerve roots that merge to form your sciatic nerve.

Herniated disk

Wear and tear or injury can cause disks to rupture (herniate), creating painful pressure on nerves.

When the disk ruptures, the rubber-like interior of the disk pokes out from its normal position between your vertebrae.

Almost everyone over age 40 has one or more bulging disks, and most people aren't bothered by them. But if the bulging material presses against an adjacent nerve, the condition can produce pain. Generally, the rupture heals over time and the pain goes away. But in some cases, nerve compression and pain can persist.

Additional causes

Other conditions that may lead to chronic back pain include:
- Joint degeneration from arthritis
- Reduced muscle tone caused by physical inactivity

Complex regional pain syndrome

Minor injury can set this painful condition off. So can a broken bone, sprain, surgical incision or any number of other injuries — usually to your hand or foot. Before long, you're experiencing a bewildering variety of painful symptoms — not only at the injury site but also in adjacent locations.

This condition used to be known as reflex sympathetic dystrophy (RSD) because it was thought to stem from an overreaction of your sympathetic nervous system, part of your autonomic nervous system that controls your heart rate, blood pressure and skin temperature. But now doctors are unsure of its cause. In fact, complex regional pain syndrome — often called CRPS — is one of the least understood forms of chronic pain.

The condition is difficult to diagnose because it's similar to other conditions. However, CRPS typically includes these unique characteristics:
- Pain that lasts longer and more intensely than you would expect from the injury
- Blood flow changes that alter the temperature, color and thickness of skin in the affected area
- Persistent swelling of the affected area

CRPS is most common in people between the ages of 40 and 60, but it can occur at any age. The pain often lasts for several months.

Fibromyalgia

Fibromyalgia is a collection of symptoms that includes widespread pain and tenderness. It differs from arthritis in that the pain is in muscles and tissues near the joints instead of in the joints themselves. Also unlike arthritis, it doesn't cause joint or muscle inflammation, nor does it destroy joints or endanger internal organs. It simply causes pain.

The main symptom of fibromyalgia is an aching all over. The pain may be a deep ache or a burning sensation. Other signs and symptoms associated with fibromyalgia may include:
- Chronic fatigue
- Digestive problems
- Difficulty sleeping
- Numbness
- Stiffness
- Tingling
- Headache
- Sensitivity to weather and temperature changes
- Pain during menstruation
- Dizziness
- Mood changes

Because these signs and symptoms commonly occur together and no specific cause has been found, fibromyalgia is referred to as a syndrome rather than a disease. In addition, because the symptoms are many and varied and don't follow a consistent pattern, fibromyalgia can be stressful as well as painful.

Most often, symptoms of fibromyalgia first become noticeable in your 30s. They may flare up and then subside, but they usually don't disappear completely. Although fibromyalgia tends to stay with you, it isn't progressive or life-threatening.

It's likely that a number of factors contribute to the development of fibromyalgia. One theory, called "central sensitization," holds that people with fibromyalgia may have a lower threshold for pain because of increased sensitivity in the brain to pain signals. Other factors may include sleep disturbances, injury, sympathetic nervous system abnormalities and changes in muscle metabolism.

Headache

Of all the pains people experience, headache is one of the most common complaints. Nearly everyone gets a headache at one time or another. Headaches can range from fleeting annoyances to those that lay you flat on your back and return often enough that they become a chronic problem. There are several types of headaches. Most fall into one of two categories.

Tension-type

This is the most common type of headache. It can range from mild to severe and can disrupt your daily routine to varying degrees. You may experience dull, tight, pressurized pain that envelopes your forehead, scalp, the back of the neck or both sides of your head. Occasionally the pain may be burning or throbbing.

Many cases of tension-type headache appear to result from contraction of the muscles on the outside of your skull. There's some evidence that enlargement of blood vessels in your scalp also may contribute to the pain. Tension-type headaches may be triggered by stressful events such as a demanding job, a bumper-to-bumper commute, or an argument with a friend or family member. Staring at a computer screen all day or other prolonged, stressful postures also can produce

tension-type headaches. These headaches can become a chronic problem.

Migraine

Up to 17 percent of women and 6 percent of men experience a more painful variety of headache known as a migraine. This type of headache not only gets your attention, it can put your life on hold.

Migraines generally produce a throbbing pain on one side of your head — often your temple or forehead. Bright lights and loud noises may intensify the pain, and you may become nauseated and vomit. The pain can range from moderate to severe. Most migraines occur for only a few hours before peaking and slowly subsiding.

Migraines were once thought to be chiefly related to blood circulation. During a migraine attack, blood vessels in your brain, neck and scalp tighten, reducing blood flow to your brain. This tightening is followed by expansion of the vessels to larger than their normal size, producing swelling and pain.

Researchers now believe these changes are a result of, and not the cause of, migraines. A more likely cause is an

Blood vessels and nerves

Migraine

A migraine appears to stem from an imbalance of brain chemicals that causes blood vessels in your brain to swell and signal pain.

imbalance of brain chemicals. Several chemicals may be related in some way to the development of migraines, including the brain chemical serotonin (ser-o-TOE-nin). During a migraine, serotonin levels generally drop.

About 10 percent of people with recurrent migraines get warning symptoms of an impending headache. These signals, called auras, often involve tingling sensations or visual distortions, such as blurred vision or zigzagging lights. They generally last less than an hour, often just 10 to 30 minutes. Migraines are thought to be hereditary, and they appear to be triggered by several factors.

Hormone fluctuations. Three times more women than men are affected by migraines. About 15 percent of women who get migraines say they occur only before, during or right after their menstrual periods. Estrogen found in birth control pills and in hormone therapy also may trigger migraine attacks in some women. For other women, their migraines diminish when taking estrogen.

Diet. Between 8 percent and 25 percent of people with migraines point to a particular food as a trigger for their attacks. The most common culprits are alcohol (especially red wine and beer), aged cheeses, chocolate, caffeine, monosodium glutamate (MSG) and fermented, pickled or marinated foods. Going too long without eating and caffeine withdrawal also can cause migraines.

Environment. Many people cite bright lights, strong odors or changes in weather conditions as triggers for their migraines.

Lifestyle. Daily stress can trigger a migraine. Migraines may also result from poor or changing sleep patterns, extreme fatigue and stress, and relief from stress.

Medications. Several medications may trigger a migraine in people who are susceptible to the headaches. They include certain high blood pressure medications, birth control pills and hormone therapy. Frequent use of a pain medication also may cause a headache when the dose wears off. This is called a rebound withdrawal headache.

Irritable bowel syndrome

Irritable bowel syndrome (IBS) — also known as functional bowel disorder — is a complex disorder in your lower intestinal tract that causes pain, bloating, gas, and recurrent bouts of diarrhea or constipation. It's a common gastro-intestinal disorder and a frequent reason people see a doctor. Fortunately, IBS doesn't result in any structural damage to the intestines.

The pain accompanying this condition often occurs below the navel, and it may be dull and aching or sharp and sudden. The condition may stem from disturbances in the nerves that control sensation or from muscle contractions in your bowel. Your central nervous system or hormonal changes also may play a role. Hormone fluctuations help explain why some women's symptoms are generally worse before or during menstruation.

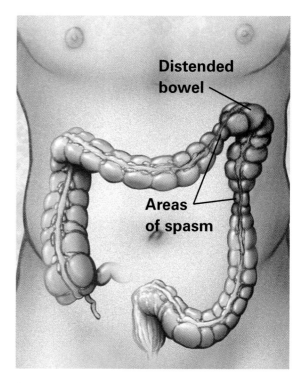

Distended bowel

Areas of spasm

Irritable bowel syndrome

A spasm in the bowel wall may cause abdominal pain and other unpleasant symptoms commonly associated with irritable bowel syndrome.

Some evidence shows that people with IBS have intestines that react more strongly to stress, activity or diet than do those in people without the condition.

There's little evidence that IBS results from particular foods. However, in some cases, fatty foods, beans and other gas-producing foods, alcohol, caffeine, and high-fiber foods may worsen symptoms.

Mouth, jaw and face pain

Some people experience chronic pain in their mouth, jaws and face (orofacial pain). Often, this pain is the result of dental problems, such as cavities or gum disease. But sometimes it can stem from other orofacial conditions.

Burning mouth syndrome

With burning mouth syndrome, you may have a burning sensation on your tongue or lips, or more widespread burning that involves your entire mouth. Burning mouth syndrome affects women seven times as often as men. It generally occurs in middle-aged or older adults. Possible causes of the condition include chronic infections, reflux of stomach acid, blood diseases, hormone imbalances and side effects of some medications. However, for many people the cause of burning mouth syndrome is unknown.

Trigeminal neuralgia

Also known as tic douloureux (doo-loo-ROO), this form of pain can develop when a blood vessel comes in contact with the trigeminal (tri-JEM-ih-nul) nerve, putting pressure on the nerve. The trigeminal nerve branches throughout your face and controls facial sensations and some muscles involved in chewing.

Trigeminal neuralgia can cause an electric shock-like pain on one side of your face and may cause you to wince as if you've been hit in the face. Jolts of pain may persist from a few seconds to a minute or two, usually returning many times a day.

Most trigeminal neuralgia pain occurs spontaneously, but the pain sometimes may be triggered by touching your face, eating, talking or brushing your teeth. Even the feeling of a breeze on your face can trigger the pain.

Trigeminal neuralgia

If you have trigeminal neuralgia, pain may occur in areas supplied by one of the three branches of the trigeminal (fifth cranial) nerve.

Temporomandibular joint

Your temporomandibular joint is where the lower jawbone connects with the skull's temporal bone. Inflammation, injury or dislocation of the joint may cause pain.

Temporomandibular disorders

The temporomandibular joints, located on each side of your face, connect your jaw to your skull. Temporomandibular joint disorders refers to a group of symptoms affecting these joints and their attached muscles.

A common symptom is pain in your jaw, face, neck or ear. Other signs and symptoms may include headaches, jaw locking or catching, and pops or clicks in your jaw during normal use.

There are several theories as to the causes of these disorders. They include trauma to the joints, degeneration of the joints and disturbance of the muscles surrounding the joints.

Other causes

Orofacial pain can also occur for other reasons that aren't well understood — and that are difficult to diagnose. Many times, the pain develops after dental treatment or a facial injury. It may be a constant aching or burning. Or it may come in the form of frequent shocks. Nerve damage in a tooth and damage to nerves in your face are other possible causes. Postherpetic neuralgia (see page 49) also can cause facial pain.

Neck pain

Similar to back pain, an injury, poor posture, or repetitive motions resulting in fatigue and overuse can strain muscles, ligaments or tendons in your neck, producing inflammation and pain. Most of the time the pain lasts for just a few days or weeks. Occasionally, though, the pain can become chronic.

Neck pain may also stem from a herniated disk or degeneration of joints in your upper spine as a result of osteoarthritis. Instead of sliding across each other smoothly, bony surfaces in your neck grate or rub on each other, producing stiffness and pain.

In addition, with age, the disks that cushion the vertebrae in your spinal column can become dry. When this occurs, the spaces in your spine where the nerves exit become narrowed and

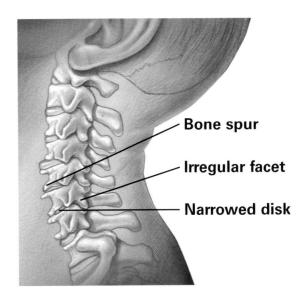

Bone spur

Irregular facet

Narrowed disk

Neck pain

Disks between bones in your neck can thin and lose elasticity. Bony outgrowths (spurs) may form. As joints rub together with greater than normal force, surfaces where they meet become irregular. Pain may result.

adjacent nerves become irritated. Other tissues and bony growths also can press on your nerves as they exit your spinal cord, causing pain.

Often, one pain leads to another. When you feel pain, you automatically tense your neck muscles to prevent further movement in a sore spot. The tension, however, also produces pain and can trigger a painful muscle spasm.

Overuse strain injuries

These injuries result from overuse of your muscles and tendons — mainly those in your hands, wrists and arms. The most noticeable symptom is pain. But an overuse injury can also cause tingling, weakness, numbness, swelling and stiffness.

Computer users, meat cutters and assembly line employees are among those commonly affected by an overuse injury. But this type of injury can occur in anyone who regularly uses repeated motions while performing daily activities.

Carpal tunnel syndrome is the most recognized overuse injury. It results from constant strain on your wrist, which can inflame the tendons located below your carpal ligament, the ligament that stretches across the palm side of your wrist. As the tendons become inflamed and swollen, they press against a nearby nerve also located beneath the carpal ligament. Pressure on this nerve is what produces the pain associated with carpal tunnel syndrome. Because the nerve runs up your arm all the way to your neck, you might feel pain anywhere along that pathway.

Most often, the result is intermittent numbness, tingling, or pain that starts in your wrist and moves down into your thumb and first two or three

Carpal ligament

Median nerve

Carpal tunnel syndrome

A narrow tunnel through your wrist (the carpal tunnel) protects your median nerve, which provides sensation to your fingers. When swelling occurs in the tunnel, the median nerve can become compressed, producing pain.

fingers. Some people find their symptoms are worse at night because of the position of their wrist or arm while sleeping. The position of your wrists when holding a book or driving a car also may trigger symptoms.

Pelvic pain

One in seven women experience some form of chronic pelvic pain. This type of pain accounts for 10 percent to 20 percent of office visits to a gynecologist. No physical cause may be found for chronic pelvic pain, but here are some known causes:

- **Endometriosis** is a condition that results when cells from the lining of a woman's uterus (endometrium) migrate into the abdominal cavity and plant themselves on structures such as the pelvic walls and surfaces of the ovaries. Some women with this condition experience pain that can be chronic. The pain is often described as a pressure-like aching in the lower abdomen.
- **Pelvic floor tension myalgia** is due to spasms of the pelvic floor muscles, which loop around the rectum and attach to the front of the pelvis.
- **Chronic pelvic inflammatory disease** (PID) can occur if a long-term infection causes your fallopian

10 tips when searching for health information on the Internet

You can find thousands of Web sites devoted to health. But — be careful. The material you'll find ranges from solid research to outright quackery. Carefully evaluate any information that you find on the Internet. Here are some suggestions when surfing the Web for information about pain or a condition you may have.

1. **Consider the source.** Any good Web site should make it easy for people to know who is responsible for the site and its information. On Mayo Clinic's Web site, for example, Mayo Clinic is clearly noted on almost every page. Look for recognized authorities such as major medical institutions and government agencies.

2. **Focus on quality.** Not all Web sites are created equal. Does the Web site have an editorial board? Is the information reviewed before it's posted? The site should identify the evidence on which the information is based and state the medical credentials of the people preparing or reviewing the information.

3. **Check for currency.** Make sure that you're getting the latest information. Look for dates on documents. Health information on Web sites should be reviewed and updated on a regular basis. Even if the information hasn't changed, you want to know it has recently been reviewed and is still valid.

4. **Be a cyberskeptic.** Does the site make health claims that seem too good to be true? Does it promise quick, dramatic and miraculous results? Does the site use obscure, scientific-sounding information? Quackery abounds on the Web. Be cautious of sites that promote "secret ingredients" or use a lot of technical jargon instead of simple language.

5. **Beware of bias.** What is the purpose of the Web site, and who is paying for it? The source of the funding can affect how the content is presented and what the individual or group is trying to accomplish. For example, is the site sponsored by a drug company and is the main purpose of the site to advertise and sell their drug? An "About This Site" link appears on many Web sites. If it's there, use it.

6. **Be cautious of chat rooms.** Chat rooms found on health information Web sites are generally developed with the intention of people sharing information about their condition or a particular problem. Some reputable sites provide chat rooms that are supervised by a health professional, but many chat rooms are unsupervised and they can become a means of passing along bad information. Chat rooms can also breed negativity — a place where people dwell on their symptoms and problems instead of trying to deal with their condition.

7. **Double-check what you're being told.** Visit several reputable Web sites and compare the information you receive. Is the advice similar or does it conflict? And remember, before you follow any medical advice, ask your doctor for guidance.

8. **Protect your privacy.** Health information should be confidential. Does the site have a privacy policy and inform you what information they collect? For example, if the site says "We share information with companies that can provide you with useful products," then your information isn't private. If there's a registration form, take note of the types of questions being asked. How is any personal information being used?

9. **Look for the HON logo.** Some Web sites post a logo from the Health On the Net (HON) Foundation. Sites that display this logo have agreed to abide by the HON Code of Conduct.

10. **Go with your gut.** If something about the site or the information you're receiving doesn't feel right, trust what your gut is telling you.

A note of caution: While it's important to be informed about your health, spending too much time reading about your condition or discussing your pain can be counterproductive. It can draw your attention to your pain, instead of away from it.

Adapted from: National Library of Medicine and the National Center for Complementary and Alternative Medicine tubes to scar and stick to your ovaries.

- **Interstitial cystitis** is a painful bladder condition that affects mainly women. It results from chronic inflammation of the bladder wall. Symptoms generally include pressure, pain and tenderness around the bladder.
- **Pelvic congestion syndrome** may be caused by varicose-type veins in various locations in the pelvis. These veins may lead to blood pooling in the ovaries and pelvic area.
- **Ovarian remnant syndrome** occurs when small pieces of ovary left behind after a hysterectomy become tiny, painful cysts.
- **Fibroids** are noncancerous uterine growths that rarely cause pain. However, they can cause pressure or a feeling of heaviness in your lower abdomen.

Peripheral neuropathy

This nerve-related condition most often affects your hands and feet, causing a tingling pain that can be accompanied by numbness. In some cases, the pain may also be shooting or burning.

Peripheral neuropathy can result from many causes, such as the side effects of medication — including some chemotherapy drugs — as well as infection or vitamin deficiencies. The most common causes are diabetes, alcoholism, autoimmune diseases such as rheumatoid arthritis or lupus, and hereditary neuropathies. There are also times when the cause of peripheral neuropathy is unclear.

The condition usually starts with a tingling sensation in your toes or the balls of your feet that spreads upward. Occasionally, it begins in your hands and extends up your arms. Numbness and weakness may follow, but the amount of pain doesn't necessarily correlate with other symptoms. Your skin also may become highly sensitive.

Postherpetic neuralgia

Postherpetic neuralgia (post-her-PET-ic noo-RAL-jah) refers to nerve damage that can occur as a result of shingles.

Shingles (herpes zoster) is caused by a reactivation of the chickenpox virus in nerve tissues. The damaged fibers aren't able to send normal pain messages. Instead, the messages become distorted and exaggerated, producing unrelenting, and often severe, pain.

Pain associated with acute shingles can take different forms, including burning, sharp and jabbing, or deep and aching. Your skin also may become hypersensitive. The slightest touch of clothing or even a change in temperature can produce a flare of pain.

Postherpetic neuralgia affects half the people older than age 60 with shingles and 75 percent of people older than age 70 with shingles. For many people, the condition gradually disappears on its own, but this can take months to several years.

Unknown causes

Sometimes, chronic pain develops for no apparent reason. Your doctor isn't able to link it to an identifiable physical cause or condition. This doesn't mean that the pain is imagined. It simply means that your pain may be associated with factors that are difficult to diagnose, or it may be due to physical processes not yet understood.

Your health is also affected by the interaction of your mind and body. For some people, psychological issues can play a role in chronic pain. For example, people who've endured sexual abuse or other kinds of physical abuse appear to have a greater risk of developing chronic pelvic or abdominal pain. It's unknown whether the pain is the result of physical injuries or if it stems from emotional scars or stress. It may be due to a combination of factors.

Chapter 4

Chronic pain cycles

People living with chronic pain often compare their lives to a roller coaster ride. There are good days when they feel uplifted and in control, followed by bad days when their mood sinks and they feel helpless. Rarely does pain stay at an even level. It fluctuates. Pain also doesn't have any boundaries. When a part of you is in pain, your whole body reacts.

As you try to understand, accept and manage your condition, your behavior and emotions may go through a series of ups and downs. This is especially true if you have debilitating pain — pain that prevents you from performing daily activities. Often, these behavioral and emotional changes follow a predictable pattern.

Behavioral cycle

One of the first noticeable effects of chronic pain is the change it brings to your regular routine. Daily tasks often become more difficult to perform, or even impossible. Here is an example of how chronic pain can easily alter your routine and behavior.

Stage 1: Decrease in activity

Because of your pain, just getting the yard rake down from its hook in the garage — much less raking the entire yard — may seem like too big of a chore. So instead, you let the leaves fall. But every time you pass by a

Behavioral cycle

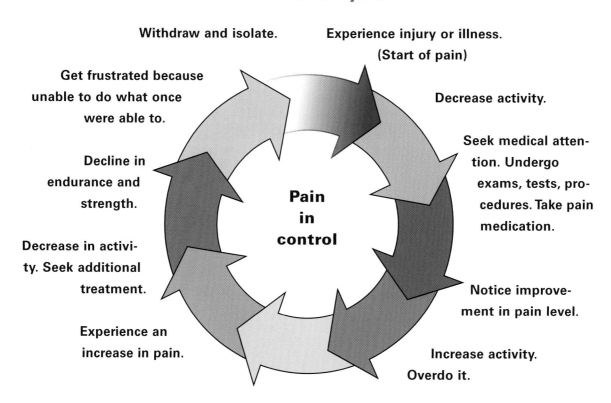

Withdraw and isolate.

Get frustrated because unable to do what once were able to.

Decline in endurance and strength.

Decrease in activity. Seek additional treatment.

Experience an increase in pain.

Experience injury or illness. (Start of pain)

Decrease activity.

Seek medical attention. Undergo exams, tests, procedures. Take pain medication.

Notice improvement in pain level.

Increase activity. Overdo it.

Pain in control

Uncontrolled chronic pain commonly causes this pattern of behavior, beginning at the top of the circle and moving clockwise.

window, you're reminded of what you can't do.

You could hire someone to rake the yard, but that would cost money. You could have your family do it, but they might feel resentful that you're not out helping them. Plus, you don't like watching others take over your responsibilities. So you wait for a day when you feel better.

Stage 2:
Increase in activity

When the day arrives that you finally feel better, you rake the yard. But you also run errands, clean the garage and go out to dinner with friends.

You put in a day best fit for a superhero. But as long as you're feeling well, why not catch up on the things you've been neglecting?

Stage 3:
More pain, less activity

The next day, you can hardly move. You feel worse than you did before your superheroic day. You chastise yourself for trying to do too much at one time and spend the next few days resting and trying to recuperate.

Eventually, you begin to feel better. But as you become more active, your pain worsens. Thinking that the only way to control your pain is to limit all physical activity, you turn over your daily chores to family and friends and spend more time in bed or on the couch.

Meanwhile, more leaves fall, friends keep calling, and you don't feel up to doing anything.

Stage 4:
Loss of strength and physical deconditioning

The time you spend lying around is making you tired, weak and less able to finish up the yardwork. Because of your long stretch of inactivity, your stamina is leaving you. You get fatigued easily. Even the thought of physical labor is daunting.

Stage 5:
Withdrawal and isolation

You find yourself spending more time alone and less time with those who care about you. Because you've stopped going out with your friends, they've stopped calling. They figure that you'd just turn them down anyway, so why bother?

Your family has gradually become accustomed to doing things without you. They now rake the yard without your help, and they've also started going out to dinner and attending social events without you. They think they're accommodating you by not forcing you to go. In response, you

Communicating your pain

When you're in pain, others can often tell it by your actions. These actions, called pain behaviors, refer to things that you do or say that let people know you're in pain. Pain behaviors are ways of calling attention to your pain — either consciously or unconsciously.

Pain behaviors are a natural response to pain. Initially, especially for acute pain, they may help reduce your pain. But over time they become ineffective. For people with chronic pain, pain behaviors often become a habit. Some common pain behaviors include:

- Limping
- Crying
- Groaning
- Grimacing
- Limiting activity
- Staying in bed
- Using protective posture
- Talking about pain, surgery or bodily functions
- Withdrawing from others

People around you generally react in one of two ways to pain behaviors: They become annoyed by them — "Not this again" — or they become overly attentive to the behaviors — "Here, let me do that." Either response creates a situation in which people tend to focus more on your illness than on you. Pain behaviors also consume a lot of energy that could be channeled into more productive ventures, such as taking steps to manage your pain.

find yourself retreating even further from your family, friends and favorite activities.

Eventually, a day comes when you begin to feel a little better. It's followed by another good day, and you begin to feel optimistic that your condition may finally be improving and you'll soon be back to your old self. But once again, your pain flares, and the cycle repeats itself.

Emotional cycle

Just as your behavior fluctuates when you're in pain, so do your emotions. Often, the two go hand in hand — the more you're able to do, the better your mood, and the less you're able to do, the worse your mood. Like your behaviors, your emotions also tend to follow a cyclic pattern.

Stage 1:
Fear and concern

When you first experience pain, you're fearful and concerned. You worry it may be a symptom of a serious disease. The more you worry, the worse it gets and the harder it becomes to ignore.

Stage 2:
Hope and promise

When you finally learn what's triggering your pain, your fear and concern are replaced with hope that your doctor will be able to make the pain disappear and your life will soon return to normal. If your doctor isn't able to find a cause, at least knowing that your pain isn't a symptom of a life-threatening condition makes you feel better.

You think that curing your pain is a reasonable request. In today's society, when something breaks we expect someone to fix it. But repairing your body is far more complicated than fixing your car or a household appliance. When the pain continues to linger despite repeated trips to various doctors, your hope starts to diminish.

In an effort to deal with your pain, you may seek to gain control in other, destructive ways, such as increasing your pain medication, drinking too much alcohol or using illicit drugs.

Stage 3:
Anger and frustration

You become dejected and depressed. This is the stage when you ask, "Why me?" and "What did I do to deserve this?" You know the pain isn't a punishment but you feel you've done something wrong, and now you're paying the price.

You may become more irritable with the people who are trying their best to help you. You may also find it easy to vent your frustration on others — your doctors, your insurance representative, and even your own family and friends.

But it's displaced anger. What's upsetting you may be the long waits at your doctor's office, the bill at the end of each visit, increased dependence on others, a sense of loss of control or, most of all, no relief from your pain.

Stage 4: Guilt and withdrawal

You feel guilty over the things you've said and done since the pain first

Overachiever's curse

Living with chronic pain isn't easy for anyone. But it can be especially difficult if you've prided yourself on being a perfectionist or you're always on the go.

If you're the sort of person who gets things done and is always called on to complete a project on time, make the cookies for the bake sale or coach the Little League team, being unable to do your part because of your pain can be devastating.

When chronic pain hits, an overachiever often has to settle for being just like everyone else. This causes some people to fall victim to all-or-nothing thinking. If they can't head the committee, they don't even want to be involved. They completely dismiss themselves from their normal activities and become withdrawn and depressed.

began. Instead of communicating this guilt, you may withdraw from people so that you won't take your anger out on them.

You also feel guilty because you aren't able to do your full share anymore. Your spouse or children have taken over some of your duties, such as par-enting responsibilities, cleaning the house or raking the yard. At work, you can't keep up your normal pace and your co-workers are having to lend you a hand. This upsets and frustrates you. But instead of venting your frustrations, you find yourself withholding your emotions and keeping them bottled up inside.

Emotional cycle

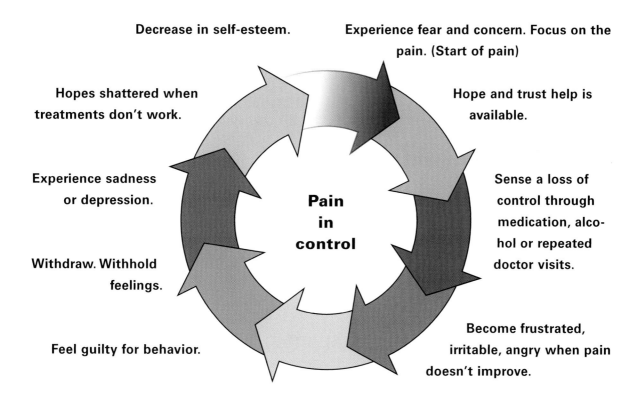

Uncontrolled chronic pain commonly causes this pattern of emotions, beginning at the top of the circle and moving clockwise.

Stage 5: Renewed hope, followed by depression

Gradually, or perhaps rather suddenly, you begin to feel better. You're optimistic that your condition is finally improving. Excitedly, you start getting back into your old routine. But after a time, the pain returns and you become deeply disappointed and lose all hope of recovery. You feel depressed and find that you can hardly make it out of bed in the morning. Things that used to matter to you, such as your appearance or attending family or social activities, don't seem important anymore.

You may begin to feel as though you're no longer loved or needed, and your self-esteem hits an all-time low. You may even begin to wonder if you're deserving of love and attention.

As you draw deeper inside yourself, your pain becomes the focus of all of your attention. Fear, isolation and depression, coupled with days of nothing to do, may make the pain feel even worse. Eventually, it becomes bad enough that it forces you to search for other forms of treatment, possibly setting you up for a repeat of the emotional cycle.

Your family's responses

Your pain, and how you react to it, don't affect just you. It also affects your family. Their responses to your behavior and emotions can take on parallel cycles of their own.

Family behaviors

When chronic pain first becomes a problem, family members generally show a great deal of support. They're often increasingly attentive to you, and they do more tasks around the house so that you can relax and "get better."

Family members also become vigilant in assessing your pain and keeping track of the activities that seem to make it better or worse. They observe and monitor you closely, in an attempt to help lessen your pain and help your doctor make a diagnosis.

When your pain doesn't improve, your family's patience may start to wear thin. They begin to resent the extra burden they've been handed. And though most family members realize that it's not your fault, it becomes

Family behavioral cycle

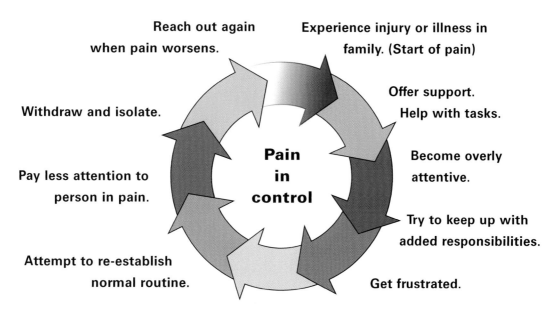

Reach out again when pain worsens.

Experience injury or illness in family. (Start of pain)

Offer support. Help with tasks.

Withdraw and isolate.

Become overly attentive.

Pay less attention to person in pain.

Try to keep up with added responsibilities.

Attempt to re-establish normal routine.

Get frustrated.

Pain in control

Family emotional cycle

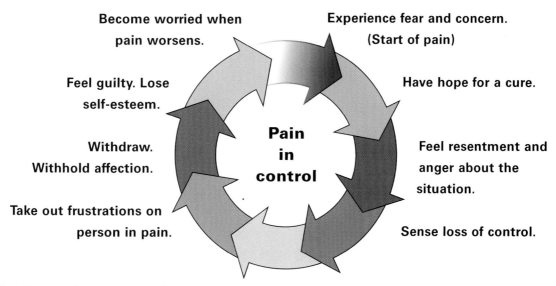

Become worried when pain worsens.

Experience fear and concern. (Start of pain)

Feel guilty. Lose self-esteem.

Have hope for a cure.

Withdraw. Withhold affection.

Feel resentment and anger about the situation.

Take out frustrations on person in pain.

Sense loss of control.

Pain in control

Family members commonly experience patterns of behavior and emotion that are similar to those of the person in pain, beginning at the top of the circle and moving clockwise.

difficult to separate the person from the pain. They may begin to withdraw and pay less attention to you.

Family emotions

Family members often go through the same emotions you do. Initially, they fear the cause of your pain. Later, when your treatment doesn't seem to be working and they're shouldering more responsibilities, they become angry and begin to ask, "Why me?" — or more appropriately, "Why us?" Just as you do, family members often feel a loss of control over their daily lives. This frustration can lead them to withhold affection because they're angry at the situation facing them. They may unintentionally take this anger out on you.

They feel bad about being angry with you and, in turn, start to feel bad about themselves and how they're acting. "I'm not a good person" and "I should be able to handle this" are common thoughts. Their guilt often leads to increased attentiveness and care, beginning the emotional cycle again.

Unfortunately, even though you and your family share common feelings, you may find these feelings difficult to talk about. Your family members fear it will sound as if they're blaming you for your pain. They also don't want to come across as being selfish and inconsiderate. The silence often brings more resentment and frustration.

Breaking the cycles

You may think that the cycles of chronic pain will never end, but you can break free of them. The downward spiral that often accompanies chronic pain occurs when all of your attention is focused on your pain.

By learning how to manage your pain, you're able to move your pain from the forefront — so that it no longer is the focus of your attention. As a result, you can concentrate on those things that give you pleasure and satisfaction. This renewed feeling will put *you* in control of your life instead of letting your pain control your life.

In upcoming chapters, we discuss a number of steps that you can take to get relief from your pain and break free from the pain cycles.

Chapter 5

Costs of chronic pain

Not everyone experiences the rippling effects of chronic pain. Some people can live with their pain without it taking a toll on their daily lives and overall health. Others aren't as lucky. If you're suffering significantly because of your pain, you're not alone.

This chapter details the personal and economic costs associated with chronic pain. It's not an upbeat discussion. But the good news is that the story doesn't end here. This book is about improving your quality of life, despite your pain. The chapters that follow this one outline what you can do to help minimize these personal and economic costs and, in some cases, avoid them.

Physical deconditioning

You know that you need regular physical activity to stay healthy. But when you're in pain, you don't feel like being active. Like many people, you may have started an exercise routine. But you did too much the first day. The next day you felt so much worse that the thought of exercising again was more than you could handle. So, you didn't. The day after, it wasn't any easier to get up and get moving, and pretty soon you found yourself doing less and less.

Inactivity generally leads to increased body fat. In addition to weight gain, having a higher proportion of body fat increases your risk of cardiovascular disease and diabetes. Inactivity can also weaken your bones and lead to a higher risk of osteoporosis. As your body becomes more deconditioned, you may begin to feel as though you may never be healthy again.

Physical activity is important to pain control. For more on the role of daily exercise in managing chronic pain, see Chapter 12.

Loss of sleep

Chronic pain reduces restful sleep. According to a Gallup Poll sponsored by the National Sleep Foundation, approximately two-thirds of people with chronic pain reported awakening too early because of their pain and being unable to fall back to sleep.

In addition to the direct effect of pain on sleep, other factors associated with chronic pain can indirectly influence how much and how well you rest:

Lack of physical activity. Inactivity makes it more difficult for you to relax and sleep well.

Excessive alcohol. Drinking too much alcohol reduces the amount of restful sleep you get at night by interfering with your brain's ability to produce adequate periods of deep sleep.

Medications. Some pain medications can stimulate your nervous system, so you don't feel tired.

When you don't get adequate sleep, you lack energy, are more easily irritated and aren't able to cope as well with pain and stress. Regular or extended bouts of sleeplessness can also wear on your health in other ways.

For more information on the association between sleep and chronic pain, as well as tips to help you sleep better, see page 212.

Emotional upheaval

Pain can play havoc with your emotions. One minute you may feel fine, the next your world may feel as though it's been torn apart. For some people, a specific event — such as an accident or fall — can change their life in an instant. For others, the development of chronic pain is a more gradual process. In either case, the pain has divided your life into two distinct parts — life as you knew it before the pain and life as you now know it with pain.

In your new life, you may feel powerless and trapped. Your emotions may range from fear and frustration to anger and apathy. Dealing with these emotions is often difficult. As you long for life before the pain, the more frustrated or angry you may become.

When you're in pain, your sense of security also may disappear. You may ask yourself: What if I lose my job? Will my family understand? What do my friends think of me? The more anxious you become, the more stressed you feel. For more on dealing with your emotions, see Chapter 14.

Depression

Depression and chronic pain often go hand in hand. Emotional strain, combined with persistent pain, creates a sinkhole that can be difficult to escape. When compared with other disorders, the prevalence of depression among people with chronic pain appears high.

It's natural to experience some discouragement when chronic pain first develops or for short periods afterward. Your pain itself may also cause symptoms, such as slowed movements or loss of energy, often associated with depression. If your symptoms linger for several months or they become severe, talk to your doctor. You may be experiencing depression.

A person with depression may have some, most or all of these symptoms:

- Lasting sadness
- Loss of interest or pleasure in most activities
- Irritability and mood swings
- Change in appetite and weight (gain or loss)
- Recurrent early awakening or other changes in sleep patterns
- Feelings of restlessness
- Feelings of hopelessness or helplessness
- Extreme fatigue, loss of energy or slowed movements
- Continual negative view of others and the world
- Feelings of worthlessness or inappropriate feelings of guilt
- Neglect of personal responsibilities and care
- Decreased concentration, attention and memory
- Decreased sex drive
- Increased focus on physical complaints
- Thoughts of death or suicide

The fundamental causes of depression aren't fully understood, but psychological and biological factors are both important. Genetic factors, imbalances in certain body or brain chemicals or abnormal sleep behaviors also may give rise to depression. In addition, living with chronic pain and having to give up enjoyable and pleasurable activities may lead to depression.

Regardless of the cause, depression is a complex condition that can make your pain feel worse. That's because it's difficult to separate your mood from your pain intensity. People who are depressed often report stronger, longer lasting and more severe pain than do people who aren't depressed.

Depression makes pain worse and should be treated. Treating depression can result in less pain or pain that's easier to manage. With treatment, up to 80 percent of people with depression show some improvement. However, many people don't receive treatment because they're unaware of their condition or they don't view depression as an illness. Treatment generally consists of cognitive behavior therapy and anti-depressant medications. These treatments are often combined.

Difficulties at work

When your first started experiencing pain, your employer may have been sympathetic to you. Perhaps your boss made your workload lighter to accommodate you, or your co-workers pitched in to help you out. But as your condition lingered, things changed. Your boss and co-workers were less willing to help you out.

Troubles with a boss or lack of understanding from co-workers can make work a stressful place. This only adds to the pain. If you're having trouble keeping up, you may also fear that you'll lose your job.

The result may be some difficult decisions. Options to control your pain and stress may include requesting a shorter workday or changing jobs. But that may not be possible or may involve some unacceptable compromises. For example, another, less stressful position may not offer a comparable salary or insurance benefits.

Financial strain

Medical bills, medications and lost days of work can strain your finances. If your pain has forced you to change or quit your job, your current income may not be sufficient to meet your expenses. To make up for the drop in income, perhaps your spouse has found a new job or is working additional hours.

Some people reach a point where they need to see a financial consultant or move to a less expensive home to avoid bankruptcy. All of these financial worries can compound your pain and further drain your sense of self-esteem.

Damaged relationships

People who were once supportive and always offering to lend a hand may not be around as much. They've gone on with their lives and seem to have less time for you.

Family relationships also seem strained. Even though your family knows you're not to blame, they're frustrated for the way your pain has changed your life and theirs.

Communication in general may be difficult. You may find yourself taking out your emotions on those closest to you. Or to the contrary, you withdraw and don't share your thoughts or feelings.

Your pain may also be straining your sexual relationship. Some people experience sexual difficulties due to pain, stress or medications. Others avoid intimacy and sexual intercourse because they no longer feel sexually attractive or they fear intercourse will increase their pain.

For more on managing personal relationships, see Chapter 16.

- Using alcohol or illicit drugs, including marijuana, to treat pain.

Similar to prescription medications, misuse of alcohol or illicit drugs as a way to relieve pain and daily pressures can also lead to chemical dependency. Plus, when you combine prescription medications with other drugs, including alcohol, you increase your risk of dangerous side effects. For more on drug dependence, see page 82.

Substance misuse

Reliance on medications and substances such as alcohol or illicit drugs can be a troublesome side effect of chronic pain. Some signs of substance misuse include:
- A preoccupation with taking medications
- Taking more medication than prescribed
- Use of more than one doctor or pharmacy to get medication
- Hiding medications or being secretive about their use
- Using someone else's medication
- Frequent use of an emergency room to get medication

Taking it one step at a time

Overcoming the costs of your pain may seem daunting. But remember that the problems that chronic pain can produce are often linked. And even a few small steps can bring noticeable results. For example, making an effort to reduce daily stress can have a positive effect on your physical health, sleep, work, personal relationships, finances and depression. As you begin to see improvements, the challenges ahead may seem less daunting.

Treating chronic pain

Chapter 6

Medication

Advances in medicine and technology have created a wide range of options for treating chronic pain. The most common form of treatment, however, remains medication. When used appropriately, medications can help reduce pain, and some people experience only limited side effects from their use. Medications can also help control a temporary flare in your pain. In addition, medications may be prescribed to help treat other conditions that can accompany chronic pain, such as depression, anxiety and sleep problems.

This chapter examines the role of medications in treating chronic pain. It also offers suggestions on how to get the most from your medications. You'll find information about specific types of drugs to treat pain, including:

- Simple pain relievers
- Opioids (narcotics)
- Topical medications
- Other pain medications
- Medications for emotional symptoms
- Medications for other physical conditions

About pain medications

The role of medications in treating chronic pain is complex and sometimes controversial. There are many kinds of medications, and doctors have varying opinions about them and how they should be used.

In part, the controversy results from the very nature of chronic pain. Treating persistent pain can be more difficult than treating acute pain, which is often a short-term condition with a clear cause.

To prescribe medications that effectively help with chronic pain, your doctor has to consider and balance a number of factors. Knowing what these factors are may help you better understand your treatment plan:

- **Rehabilitation.** Treatment of chronic pain shouldn't simply aim at controlling symptoms. The larger goal is to help you lead a full and active life.

- **Efficacy.** This term refers to the power of a medication to produce desired results — in this case, a reduction in the level of pain. Higher doses of a medication may not increase its efficacy. In fact, a higher dose may increase the risk of side effects.

- **Safety.** Pain medications can cause side effects such as stomach bleeding and liver damage. Over the short term, you may be able to tolerate side effects. However, when medication is used for weeks or months, the risk of side effects becomes a larger issue.

- **Interactions.** Your doctor will try to avoid drug combinations that cause unsafe interactions — unwanted effects that can occur when some drugs are taken together. Equally important is preventing drug-disease interactions — prescribing a drug for chronic pain that may worsen another condition, such as diabetes. Finally, interactions with over-the-counter medications, alcohol and certain foods also may cause problems.

- **Allergies.** An allergy to one pain medication may eliminate an entire class of drugs that could be used in your treatment.

- **Life setting.** To understand this factor, compare two people. One is an older adult who has high levels of pain due to an end-stage cancer. Another is a middle-aged person with chronic back pain who still maintains a full work and family life. The person with cancer may have a treatment plan that calls for higher doses of medication to deliver immediate pain relief. The second person may need to balance dosage and pain relief with safety and ability to function in daily life.

- **Placebo effects.** If you try a new pain medication, you might feel better at first, even though the new medication has no specific advantage over a previously used medication. This is the placebo effect, and

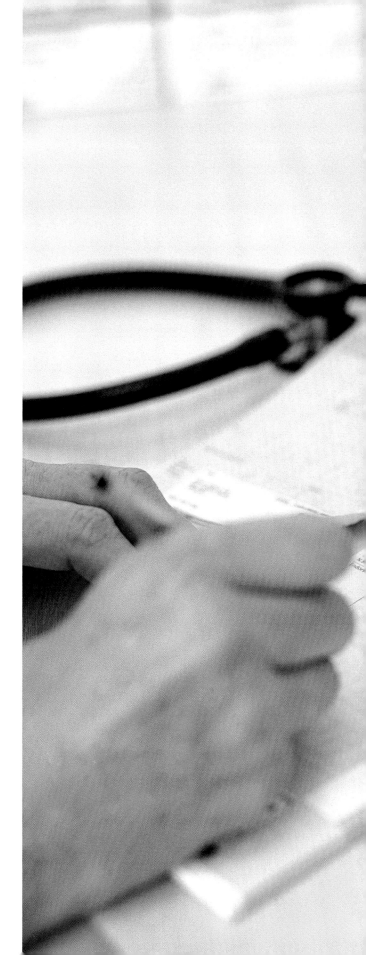

it can complicate treatment for chronic pain.

- **Practical issues.** You and your doctor also need to consider the cost of your medication and the challenges of sticking to a medication schedule. Some pain medications are short acting and must be taken several times a day. Other medications have longer lasting effects and can be taken less often.

In light of these factors, your doctor likely will want to tailor your medication to your specific needs and circumstances, applying the concept of hierarchical treatment. This means that your treatment may take place in stages. You may begin with fewer medications in lower doses with fewer potential side effects. You and your doctor will judge how well this approach works before trying stronger medications, adding to the number of medications, increasing doses or risking more side effects.

Remember that medication is usually just one option in a full treatment plan. Your plan may also include physical therapy, counseling and lifestyle changes. Some people find these other therapies help reduce or eliminate their need for pain medication.

Wise use of medications

One of the most important things you can do to get the most from your medication is to be actively involved in your care. The following steps can increase the safety and efficacy of your medications.

Share information

Your doctor needs to know exactly which medications you take. Keep an up-to-date list of all of your medications — including what you take to relieve pain — or keep your medications in their original containers and bring them along when you see your doctor. Include both prescription and nonprescription medications, as well as dietary supplements and herbs. Know these details:

- **Name of medication.** To avoid confusion, remember that medications have both generic and brand names.

- **Dosage.** Dosage refers to the amount of medication you take at one time and how often you take the medication.

- **Purpose.** Why did you begin taking the medication? For example, was it prescribed to treat your pain or to treat a condition associated with your pain, such as insomnia or depression?

- **How you take the medication.** Do you take the medication with or without food? Do you take it just before going to bed or earlier in the day?

- **Results.** Do you feel any unexpected side effects from the medication? How well do you think the drug is working?

- **Other health conditions.** If you're allergic to certain medications or think you might be pregnant, be sure to tell your doctor. Also mention any other illnesses or conditions you have.

Be informed

Keep and read the printed materials that come with your medications. These materials offer general information that may answer some of your questions. Make sure you know exactly why you're taking the medication and what results you can expect.

Stick to your plan

Take your medication exactly as prescribed. If you stop taking a drug before your prescription ends, you could undermine your treatment results. The same thing can happen if you cut down on a medication without consulting your doctor or if you take more than prescribed.

Speak up

Medication that worked well for you several months or years ago could have different effects on you today. Sometimes doses need to be changed or the whole treatment plan needs to be adjusted. Carefully observe day-to-day changes in your health and report those changes to your doctor.

Simple pain relievers

Simple pain relievers, also called analgesics (an-ul-JE-ziks), are medications designed to reduce or relieve pain. They control pain in various ways by interfering with the processes in which pain messages are developed, transmitted or interpreted. Simple analgesics

are different from narcotic medications — also known as opioids — described later in this chapter.

Acetaminophen

Acetaminophen includes the brand-name drug Tylenol. It's most effective for mild to moderate pain that isn't accompanied by inflammation.

When taken occasionally and as recommended, acetaminophen is safe. The drug is generally considered less problematic than other simple pain relievers because it doesn't cause side effects such as stomach pain and bleeding. However, if you frequently take more acetaminophen than recommended on the product label, you risk liver or kidney damage. Taking acetaminophen with alcohol also increases that risk and can lead to sudden and severe problems such as liver failure. In addition, unlike other pain relievers, acetaminophen does little to reduce inflammation.

Acetaminophen is sometimes combined with an opioid to provide stronger pain relief. These drugs are available only by prescription. Whenever you use a combination of medications, ask your doctor or pharmacist about the use and side effects of each drug.

Nonsteroidal anti-inflammatory drugs

Nonsteroidal anti-inflammatory drugs (NSAIDs) are most effective for mild to moderate pain that's accompanied by swelling and inflammation. They relieve pain by inhibiting an enzyme in your body called cyclooxygenase (si-klo-OX-suh-juhn-ays). This enzyme makes hormone-like substances called prostaglandins, involved in the development of pain and inflammation.

NSAIDs are especially helpful for arthritis and pain resulting from muscle sprains, strains, back and neck injuries, or cramps.

There are several brands of NSAIDs sold by prescription. Nonprescription NSAIDs available over-the-counter include:

- Aspirin
- Ibuprofen (Advil, Motrin, others)
- Naproxen sodium (Aleve)

When taken as directed, NSAIDs are generally safe. But if you take more than the recommended dosage — and sometimes even the recommended dosage — NSAIDs may cause nausea, stomach pain, stomach bleeding or ulcers. Large doses of NSAIDs can also lead to kidney problems, fluid retention and high blood pressure. Risk of these conditions increases with age. If you regularly take NSAIDs, talk to your doctor so that he or she can monitor you for side effects.

NSAIDs also have a so-called ceiling effect — a limit as to how much pain they can control. This means that beyond a certain dosage, they don't provide additional benefit. If you have moderate to severe pain, exceeding the dosage recommendations may not help to relieve your pain.

COX-2 inhibitors

This class of medications is similar to NSAIDs, but the drugs work in a

Peripheral nerves

Normal knee

Osteoarthritic
knee

NSAIDs

NSAIDs reduce the chemicals that sensitize peripheral nerves, causing the nerves
to send out pain signals. NSAIDs are often
used to reduce pain associated with
inflammatory diseases and conditions,
such as arthritis and muscle sprains.

different manner. COX-2 inhibitors were developed with the aim of reducing some of the well-recognized side effects of traditional NSAIDs. But COX-2 inhibitors appear to be associated with an increased risk of cardiovascular problems. For this reason, several of these drugs have been withdrawn from the market and currently only one COX-2 inhibitor remains — the drug celecoxib (Celebrex).

Like traditional NSAIDs, COX-2 inhibitors block production of the enzyme cyclooxygenase (COX). But unlike traditional NSAIDs, they affect only one form of the enzyme.

Cyclooxygenase comes in two forms — COX-1 and COX-2. Part of the role of COX-1 is to protect your stomach lining. Because NSAIDs suppress the function of COX-1, side effects such as stomach pain and bleeding problems can result. COX-2 inhibitors affect only COX-2, the form of the enzyme involved in the development of inflammation. Therefore, they cause fewer digestive problems.

However, COX-2 inhibitors can still produce side effects, including symptoms of respiratory infection, headache and dizziness. And although the risk of

stomach bleeding is generally lower if you take a COX-2 inhibitor instead of an NSAID, bleeding can still occur. In addition, these drugs can lead to kidney problems, fluid retention and high blood pressure. Older adults may be at higher risk of all of these side effects.

With both COX-2 inhibitors and traditional NSAIDs, the goal is to take the lowest effective dose for the shortest duration possible.

Opioids (narcotics)

Opioids, commonly called narcotics, are prescription medications that are regulated as controlled substances by the Drug Enforcement Administration. A doctor must have a special license in order to prescribe these medications.

Opioids are often used to relieve pain from cancer, terminal illness, severe injury or surgery. Pain control after surgery is especially important because the sooner you're active, the less your risk of complications that can follow surgery, such as pneumonia or blood clots, caused by inactivity.

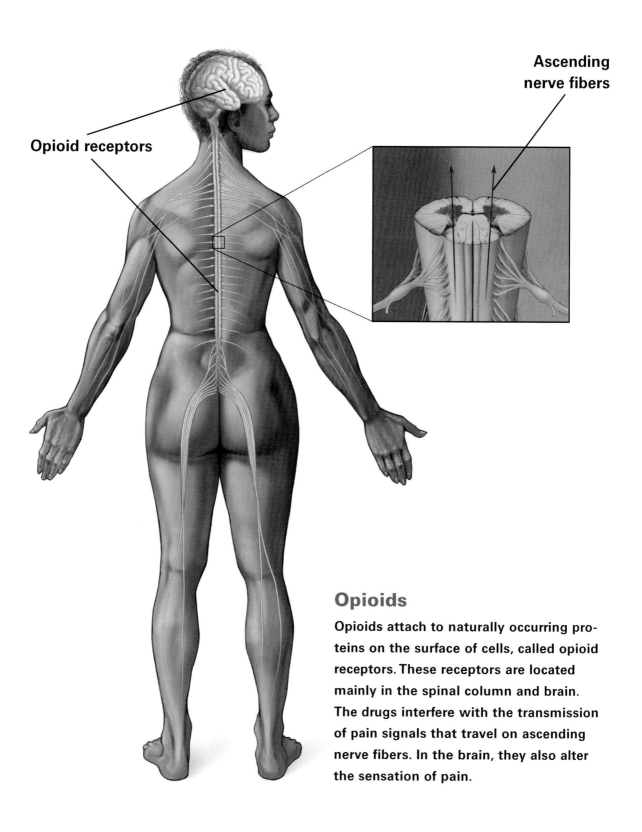

Opioid receptors

Ascending nerve fibers

Opioids

Opioids attach to naturally occurring proteins on the surface of cells, called opioid receptors. These receptors are located mainly in the spinal column and brain. The drugs interfere with the transmission of pain signals that travel on ascending nerve fibers. In the brain, they also alter the sensation of pain.

Opioids come in several forms. Some are natural compounds derived from the opium poppy plant. These compounds are called opiates. There are also synthetic opioids that work in similar ways. The term *opioids* refers to both natural and synthetic forms of the drug.

Most opioids are agonists, a drug that binds to a receptor of a cell and triggers a response by the cell. An agonist produces an action, whereas an antagonist acts against, or blocks, an action. Some opioid pain relievers are mixed agonists and antagonists — they work in two ways to relieve pain. Examples of mixed opioids include the drugs buprenorphine (Buprenex, Subutex), butorphanol (Stadol), levorphanol (Levo-Dromoran), nalbuphine (Nubain) and pentazocine (Talwin).

Opioid agonists, meanwhile, include:
- Codeine
- Fentanyl (Duragesic)
- Hydrocodone plus acetaminophen (Vicodin, Lortab)
- Hydromorphone (Dilaudid)
- Meperidine (Demerol)
- Methadone (Dolophine)
- Morphine (MS Contin, Oramorph SR, others)

- Oxycodone (OxyContin)
- Oxymorphone (Numorphan)
- Propoxyphene (Darvon)

Side effects of opioids — particularly when they're taken at higher doses — include mild dizziness, drowsiness, sedation and unclear thinking. These can make it unsafe for you to drive or operate machinery. Sometimes you can do things to manage the dizziness. For example, you might feel better after lying down for a while. If you experience severe dizziness or drowsiness, get emergency care. Also go to the emergency room if you feel extreme nervousness, experience severe weakness, have cold and clammy skin or have trouble breathing.

Other side effects of the medications include fatigue, constipation, nausea and vomiting. Ask your doctor or pharmacist about ways to manage these. In addition, opioids can lead to physical dependence or addiction (see page 82).

The debate over opioid use

With acute pain, the goal is to treat and relieve pain as quickly as possible, usually with medications. Unrelieved pain

Understanding the risk of addiction

The issue of addiction is important, especially if you're taking an opioid (narcotic) medication. Many discussions about the effects of opioids get confused because people use three terms synonymously: tolerance, physical dependence and addiction. These words actually refer to three different conditions:

- **Tolerance** happens when the initial dose of a narcotic loses its effectiveness over time. Some people refer to this as becoming "immune" to the drug. To get the same pain-relieving effect, you need to take higher doses of the medication. Unfortunately, in many cases, increasing the dose of the drug results in increased or unacceptable side effects.

- **Physical dependence** occurs when your body becomes accustomed to a drug. When the drug is withdrawn, you may experience anxiety, tremors and other physical withdrawal symptoms.

- **Addiction** is the term used to identify the irresistible craving for, loss of control over the use of, compulsive use of and continued use of a drug, despite repeated, harmful consequences. Drugs capable of producing addiction do so by interacting with the biochemistry of the brain in such a way that the drug seems essential — you feel the "need" for it just as you do food and water.

With time, people who take a narcotic are likely to develop tolerance and even physical dependence. However, this doesn't mean that they are, or will become, addicted to the drug. Most people treated with narcotics never experience addiction. Addiction results from many factors — genetic, psychological and environmental — and it often takes years to develop. Use of the drug is only one factor.

Sometimes, people with chronic pain act in ways that are mistakenly called addictive. These people may focus on maintaining their supply of opioids or closely watch the clock to make sure they take their next dose of medication. Often these are not addictive behaviors but pseudoaddiction — behaviors that stop once people get satisfactory pain relief.

has many negative effects, such as delayed recovery from surgery and decreased immunity to disease.

For people with chronic pain, the goals of treatment are more complex. Pain relief is important, but so is the ability to function at work and to be able to enjoy social and leisure activities.

Sometimes, the goal of pain relief comes into conflict with the goal of improved physical functioning — especially when it comes to the use of opioids. Opioids are powerful pain relievers. When taken in small amounts and for short periods, they generally cause only minor side effects. But when opioids are taken in increasing doses for several weeks or months, these side effects can impair your ability to function.

Opioids can also have an effect described as rebound pain. For instance, the effects of some opioids last only a few hours. Pain can recur as these short-acting medications wear off or when they're withdrawn from your treatment plan.

Opioids can also cause changes in your nervous system that actually may heighten your perception of pain and make you feel more uncomfortable. This condition is called hyperalgesia.

In summary, opioids have many effects, some good and others not so good. For this reason — in addition to the fact that opioids aren't effective for all types of pain — some doctors prefer not to use opioids when treating chronic pain. They may also be uneasy about the possible long-term side effects of opioids, which can interfere with rehabilitation and lead to more doctor visits and hospital stays. Doctors also cite the risk of physical dependence and addiction to the drugs.

Other doctors, meanwhile, take the position that withholding opioids leads to unnecessary pain and suffering, that the side effects of opioids can be managed, and that the risk of addiction is overblown. This view of opioids holds that legal and medically supervised use of the medications has little in common with illegal use of such drugs.

Opioids as part of your pain treatment plan

Although there's debate over the use of narcotics, these medications can be a key part of your treatment plan if your doctor feels they can reduce your pain without causing severe side effects. Before prescribing the drugs, your doctor likely will get a detailed medical history and have you undergo a thorough physical exam. The results can help determine whether opioids are right for you.

Consider your full range of options if taking a narcotic. Ask about the possibility of combining an opioid with a simple analgesic for maximum pain relief. Compare the benefits of short-acting and sustained-release medications. Discuss whether you should take the medications on a regular schedule or simply on an as-needed basis. You may also want to get a second opinion.

Finally, compare your function and activity levels with how you were functioning before you started the medication. If you haven't seen a marked improvement, you may not want to continue using the drug.

Topical medications

Topical medications are products that are applied to the skin to help relieve pain. These drugs act on the surface of your body or are absorbed through the skin where they may help relieve nerve pain and inflammation just below the skin's surface.

Local anesthetics

Local anesthetics inhibit pain signals along nerves at the site where the medication is applied. They're sold as patches, gels and creams.

Lidocaine patch. A lidocaine patch (Lidoderm) may be prescribed for relief of pain associated with postherpetic neuralgia and nerve pain. Redness and swelling may occur at the application site.

Nonprescription products. There are several topical medications available without a prescription for pain relief. They include lidocaine (Xylocaine, Zilactin-L), benzocaine (Lanacane) and pramoxine (Prax, Itch-X).

Other analgesics

Other topical medications used to treat pain include the following:

Ketamine-amitriptyline cream. This product is a combination of the medications ketamine and amitriptyline.

The cream is used most often for nerve-related (neuropathic) pain, including pain and tingling in the feet and hands (peripheral neuropathy) associated with diabetes. It's available only by prescription.

Capsaicin. This nonprescription drug is made from the seeds of hot chili peppers. It's thought to work by depleting nerve cells of a chemical called substance P, which has a role in transmitting pain messages.

You rub capsaicin (Capzasin-P, Zostrix) on your skin, typically three or five times a day. It usually takes up to two weeks before you begin to feel noticeable pain relief. Some people find capsaicin effective for temporary relief of arthritic pain in joints close to your skin's surface, such as your fingers, knees and elbows. It may also help relieve pain after shingles (postherpetic neuralgia). However, it can temporarily

irritate your skin and produce a burning sensation, which is painful in and of itself.

Trolamine salicylate. Medications such as Aspercreme and Sportscreme contain a chemical that's similar to aspirin called trolamine salicylate. This chemical decreases the ability of nerve endings in the skin to sense pain. The Food and Drug Administration (FDA) lists products containing trolamine salicylate as safe, but not necessarily effective for pain relief. They're available without a prescription.

Counterirritant products

These nonprescription preparations (ArthriCare, Bengay, Icy Hot) stimulate nerve endings in the skin to produce feelings of cold, warmth or itching. These responses — which may be mildly painful — counter, or block, more intense pain sensations.

Counterirritant products may relieve occasional, mild muscle aches and joint pain — simple strains and sprains — but they're generally not effective for most forms of chronic pain. In addition, they typically require frequent applications, and some products have a medicinal smell.

Other pain medications

Additional medications commonly used to treat chronic pain include drugs that work similarly to narcotics but aren't true opioids, as well as drugs developed for other conditions that have been found to be effective in relieving some types of pain.

Tramadol

Tramadol (Ultram) is a prescription pain medication that's used mainly to relieve mild to moderate pain. It works in two ways. Though the drug isn't an opioid (narcotic), it works like one in that it interferes with the transmission of pain signals. It also affects certain brain chemicals (neurotransmitters) to decrease the perception of pain.

Because tramadol isn't a true opioid, risk of physical dependence and addiction is less. However, the drug isn't completely free of these risks. More common side effects can include dizziness, sedation, headache, nausea, constipation and seizures. Tramadol is also available in an extended-release form and in combination with aceta-minophen. The combination drug is called Ultracet.

Tricyclic antidepressants

Tricyclic antidepressants are a class of antidepressants that are also used to treat chronic pain. In addition to relieving symptoms of depression, tricyclic antidepressants interfere with certain chemical processes that cause you to feel pain. The drugs appear to strengthen the system that inhibits, or blocks, pain messages.

Tricyclic antidepressants commonly used to manage pain include the medications:
- Amitriptyline
- Clomipramine (Anafranil)
- Desipramine (Norpramin)
- Doxepin (Sinequan)
- Imipramine (Tofranil)
- Nortriptyline (Pamelor)
- Protriptyline (Vivactil)
- Trimipramine (Surmontil)

Antidepressants don't cause dependence or addiction. However, tricyclic antidepressants can make you drowsy. Therefore, it's generally recommended that you take the medication in the evening before bed. In addition, these drugs may cause dry mouth, blurred

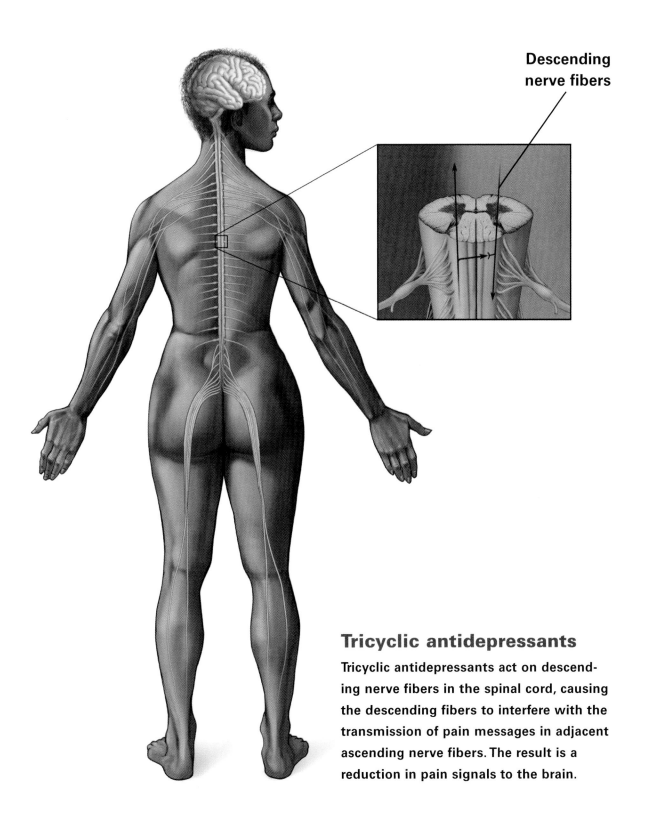

Descending nerve fibers

Tricyclic antidepressants

Tricyclic antidepressants act on descending nerve fibers in the spinal cord, causing the descending fibers to interfere with the transmission of pain messages in adjacent ascending nerve fibers. The result is a reduction in pain signals to the brain.

vision, constipation, difficulty with urination, weight gain, changes in blood pressure and confusion. Side effects usually begin soon after you start taking the medication or your dose is increased, but pain relief may not occur for several weeks. Tricyclic antidepressants can also interfere with cardiac conduction, the manner and rate at which the heart produces electrical impulses.

To reduce or prevent these symptoms, your doctor will likely start you off at a low dose and slowly increase the amount. Most people are able to take tricyclic antidepressants, particularly in low doses, with only mild side effects.

Serotonin and norepinephrine reuptake inhibitors (SNRIs)

This class of medications includes the drug duloxetine (Cymbalta). Duloxetine is an antidepressant that's sometimes prescribed to relieve pain caused by nerve damage in people with diabetes (diabetic neuropathy). The drug is thought to control pain by enhancing nerve signals within the central nervous system that naturally inhibit pain messages. Possible side effects include constipation, dizziness,

drowsiness, sleep problems, stomach pain, nausea and loss of appetite.

Anti-seizure medications

Several drugs developed primarily to control or reduce epileptic seizures have been found to help certain pain conditions, primarily the stabbing or shooting pain resulting from nerve damage. The drugs seem to work by quieting damaged nerves to slow or prevent uncontrolled pain signals.

Anti-seizure medications that may be used to treat chronic pain include:
- Carbamazepine (Carbatrol, Tegretol)
- Divalproex sodium (Depakote)
- Gabapentin (Neurontin)
- Lamotrigine (Lamictal)
- Levetiracetam (Keppra)
- Phenytoin (Dilantin)
- Oxcarbazepine (Trileptal)
- Pregabalin (Lyrica)
- Tiagabine (Gabitril)
- Topiramate (Topamax)

These medications can cause dizziness, drowsiness, nausea and lack of balance and coordination, short-term memory disturbance, and weight gain. But, again, most people are bothered only minimally. More severe but less

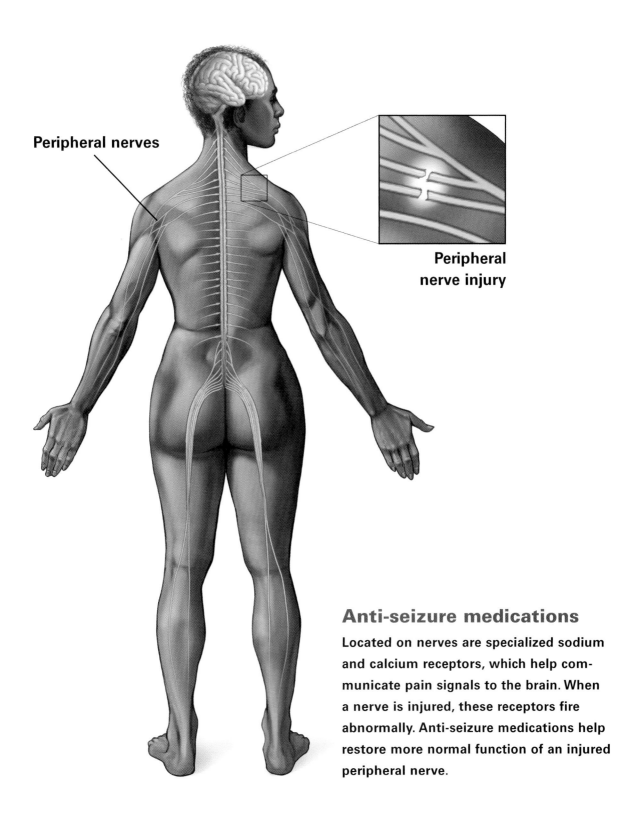

Peripheral nerves

Peripheral nerve injury

Anti-seizure medications

Located on nerves are specialized sodium and calcium receptors, which help communicate pain signals to the brain. When a nerve is injured, these receptors fire abnormally. Anti-seizure medications help restore more normal function of an injured peripheral nerve.

common side effects include skin, blood and liver disorders. To reduce your risk of side effects, your doctor will likely start you off on a small amount of the drug and gradually increase the dose.

Emotional symptoms

In addition to relieving your pain, there are other reasons that your doctor may prescribe medication. The intent of these drugs isn't to reduce your pain but to relieve other troubling symptoms associated with chronic pain. This is important because when you're not bothered by other symptoms, you can direct more of your energy toward your daily activities.

Depression and anxiety

Depression and anxiety are common among people who have chronic pain. Relief from these conditions can have a significant effect on your ability to manage your pain. That's because as you begin to feel better — more energetic and more in control — your pain seems more tolerable and manageable.

Experts believe depression results from an imbalance in certain brain chemicals (neurotransmitters) that affect your mood and emotions. The condition is often treated with medications that increase production of these chemicals. Anxiety is also thought to result from a combination of biochemical changes, and is treated with many of the same medications as depression.

In addition to tricyclic antidepressants, discussed earlier, other types of medications used to treat depression and anxiety include:

Selective serotonin reuptake inhibitors (SSRIs). These medications have become a first line treatment for depression and anxiety because they produce few serious side effects. The drugs influence the activity of certain brain chemicals, helping nerve cells in your brain send and receive messages. SSRIs include the medications:

- Citalopram (Celexa)
- Escitalopram (Lexapro)
- Fluoxetine (Prozac, Sarafem)
- Paroxetine (Paxil)
- Sertraline (Zoloft)

SSRIs don't work immediately. It may take up to eight weeks before you experience the full effects of the drugs.

Buying medications online: The do's and don'ts

Ordering prescription drugs online can save you time and sometimes even money. But you must be careful. Questionable online pharmacies may ship expired drugs or those that haven't been stored properly. Others don't require a prescription or check for drug interactions. To safeguard your health and finances, remember these simple do's and don'ts.

Do:
- *Consult your doctor.* Your doctor can determine if it's OK to purchase your medication from an online site and also provide advice on cautions to be aware of, should you decide to do so.
- *Use a licensed pharmacy.* The National Association of Boards of Pharmacy can tell you whether a particular online pharmacy is licensed and in good standing.
- *Insist on access to a registered pharmacist.* Reputable sites offer toll-free access to registered pharmacists who can help answer your medication questions.
- *Read the privacy and security policies.* Before placing an order, be confident that your credit card number, personal health information and other personally identifiable information will be protected.
- *Be cautious of sites based in foreign countries.* Legitimate international sites exist. But there are risks. The medication may not be held to the same rigorous safety standards as in the United States.

Don't:
- *Use a site that bypasses prescriptions.* Only your doctor can safely prescribe medication.
- *Order medication that's not approved by the Food and Drug Administration.* Taking an inappropriate or unsafe drug may have life-threatening consequences.
- *Succumb to false claims.* Don't buy medication from sites that advertise "miracle cures" or those that use impressive terminology to disguise a lack of good science.

They also can cause some side effects. Up to 30 percent of people experience sexual problems. However, once you stop taking the drug, the problems usually go away. Other side effects may include headache, dizziness, nausea and diarrhea.

Other antidepressants. These medications are prescribed mainly for the treatment of anxiety. They work similarly to SSRIs but affect different brain chemicals:

- Bupropion (Wellbutrin)
- Mirtazapine (Remeron)
- Venlafaxine (Effexor)

Anxiolytics. Anxiolytics are a form of benzodiazepines that reduce feelings of anxiety. They differ from other types of benzodiazepines developed to act as sedatives and help promote drowsiness. Anxiolytics include the medications:

- Alprazolam (Xanax)
- Clonazepam (Klonopin)
- Diazepam (Valium)
- Lorazepam (Ativan)

Anxiolytics can become habit-forming if you take them for more than a few weeks. Your doctor may prescribe the medication only for a short time to get you through an anxious period.

Buspirone (BuSpar). This is an anti-anxiety medication that works by stimulating serotonin receptors on nerves, altering the chemical messages that nerves transmit to each other. Unlike some other anti-anxiety medications, buspirone doesn't cause sedation. However, it takes a couple of weeks for the effects of the drug to become noticeable. Buspirone is most effective for mild to moderate anxiety symptoms. Side effects may include dizziness, headache, nausea and insomnia.

Sleep disturbance

Pain affects sleep. If you're in pain, you may have trouble falling asleep or your pain may wake you up at night and you may not be able to get back to sleep. Just the opposite, the medication you're taking for your pain may make you drowsy and cause too much sleep.

A good night's sleep is important because it can help you better cope with your pain by renewing your energy level and improving your mood. Medications prescribed to promote sleep include:

Antidepressants. Drowsiness is a common side effect of some antidepressants. When taken at night before bed, the drugs may help you sleep better — in addition to controlling pain and depression. The antidepressant trazodone (Desyrel) is commonly prescribed to help improve sleep.

Sedatives. Sedatives help promote sleep. However, they can cloud your thinking, make you drowsy, impair your balance and affect your ability to drive. If taken for more than just a short period, some sedatives may also cause dependency or addiction.

Sedatives can be divided into two broad categories — benzodiazepines and nonbenzodiazepines. Benzodiazepines are an older class of sleeping pills. They're more likely to cause headache and drowsiness in the morning and they can be habit-forming. Benzodiazepines include:

- Estazolam (ProSom)
- Temazepam (Restoril)
- Triazolam (Halcion)

Nonbenzodiazepines include the newest class of sleeping pills. These drugs induce sleep by quieting the nervous system. They're metabolized more quickly, which helps reduce the risk of side effects the next day. Commonly used nonbenzodiazepines include:

- Eszopiclone (Lunesta)
- Ramelteon (Rozerem)
- Zaleplon (Sonata)
- Zolpidem (Ambien)

Sleeping pills are a temporary solution for sleep problems while other efforts to improve sleep have time to work. They should be used for only a few nights at a time. Even newer medications aren't without potentially serious side effects. Some have been found to promote sleepwalking in which people get out of bed and perform tasks or activities during the night that they have no recollection of in the morning.

Related physical conditions

Sometimes, chronic pain is associated with other physical conditions that also need to be addressed in order for pain relief treatments to be effective.

Muscle spasms

If your pain is accompanied by muscle spasms, your doctor may recommend a muscle relaxant to control the spasms. Muscle relaxants are best used on a short-term, as-needed basis — a period of three to five days — because they can cause side effects. For example, the drugs can cloud your thinking and leave you drowsy and dizzy, especially when taken in combination with an opioid (narcotic). Muscle relaxants include these prescription drugs:

- Carisoprodol (Soma)
- Cyclobenzaprine (Flexeril)
- Methocarbamol (Robaxin)
- Orphenadrine (Norflex)
- Tizanidine (Zanaflex)

Inflammation

If your pain is related to rheumatoid arthritis or another inflammatory condition, your doctor may prescribe oral anti-inflammatory medications, including NSAIDs and steroids. These drugs are used both to ease the pain and to reduce inflammation that may damage your joints.

If you have an acutely inflamed joint, an NSAID may not be effective and your doctor may prescribe an oral corticosteroid. Corticosteroids may be used short term or, in some cases, long term to manage a more serious problem. Widely used corticosteroids include the oral drugs hydrocortisone and prednisone.

The benefits vs. the risks

There's no question that medications play an important role in the treatment of chronic pain, but they should be used judiciously — weighing the benefits of a particular drug against its potential for serious side effects. A drug is generally considered to be of benefit if it results in less pain, improved function and a return to everyday activities, while causing only minimal side effects.

As you consider the role of medications in controlling your pain it's important to remember that each person is different and not all people respond in the same manner to various medications. A drug that works for one person may not for you. Likewise, a drug that you find helpful may be of little benefit to someone else.

Don't make judgments simply on what you read or hear about medications. The best place to get advice is from your doctor or other health care provider who is helping you to manage your pain.

Chapter 7

Injections, stimulators and pumps

W hen it comes to methods to relieve pain, the first thing most people think of is medication. However, there are several ways to treat chronic pain beyond oral medications. Options range from using needles to inject medication at or near the site of the pain, to implanting pain-relieving devices in your body, such as nerve stimulators and medication pumps. Depending on the type of pain you have and its severity, one of these approaches may work for you.

Injection therapy

Instead of prescribing pills to control the pain, your doctor might inject medication at or near the pain site to see if it can provide pain relief. Injections generally don't cure pain, but they may help you through an initial period of intense pain or a flare-up of severe pain.

Injections are most effective for joint, muscle or nerve pain that's confined to a specific location. The type of drug injected may be an anesthetic to control the pain, a steroid to reduce inflammation or a combination of the two.

One benefit of injections is that the medication works primarily, but not exclusively, in a limited part of your body. By targeting a specific area, injections may reduce the amount of medication needed as well as the number and intensity of side effects.

In addition to providing pain relief, injections may be used to help diagnose the cause of your pain. Suppose, for example, that a small amount of anesthetic injected at a specific location relieves your pain. This indicates that a particular joint, muscle or nerve may be the source of the pain. Once your doctor knows the pain source, it's possible he or she can find more effective methods to treat it.

In deciding whether injections may be right for you, keep in mind that you'll have to visit your doctor's office for each procedure. In addition, the site of the injection and the type of medication used can limit how often you receive an injection. For instance, injected steroids may cause adverse side effects that become worse with frequent use. Therefore, doctors generally limit the number of injections you can have.

Injections are seldom used by themselves to treat chronic pain. They're generally most effective when given in conjunction with a program that also includes physical therapy. Injections may make such therapy more comfortable.

The types of injections used to treat chronic pain can be divided into three broad categories: peripheral joint and nerve injections, soft tissue injections and spinal injections.

Peripheral joint and nerve injections

Peripheral injections are used to reduce pain in large, weight-bearing joints and in major peripheral nerves. Your peripheral nerves are those nerves that extend from your spinal cord into your arms and hands and your legs and feet.

Your peripheral joints include your hip and knee joints, and other large joints such as your shoulder and elbow joints. When these joints become inflamed and painful, your doctor may inject medications into them to ease your discomfort. Peripheral joint injections can provide immediate pain relief, giving other methods to control the pain, such as physical therapy or oral medications, time to work.

Peripheral nerve injections work in the same way, but instead of the medication being injected into a joint, it's injected around a specific group of nerves. This temporarily prevents pain messages that are traveling along that nerve pathway from reaching your brain.

In addition to helping manage pain, peripheral nerve injections are also used to help diagnose the source of pain. If a medication injected near a specific nerve eliminates or significantly reduces your pain, doctors know that nerve is likely the source of your pain.

Commonly targeted nerves include:
- **Intercostal nerves.** These nerves lie between the ribs. An intercostal injection may be used to help control pain from an injured nerve in the rib area.

- **Occipital nerves.** The occipital nerves provide sensation to the

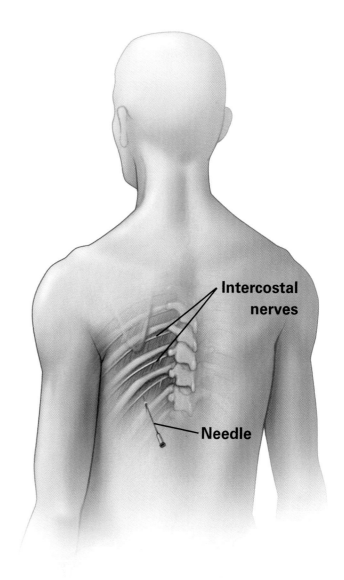

Intercostal injection

An intercostal injection blocks the transmission of pain signals in the intercostal nerves, which originate in the spinal cord and run under the ribs.

back of the neck and head. An occipital injection is given at the base of the skull or back of the neck. It may be used in the diagnosis or treatment of conditions such as headache or chronic jaw pain.

- **Large peripheral nerves.** With this type of injection, medication is placed in the area surrounding a large peripheral nerve, such as the femoral nerve, the major nerve that runs from your spine down each of your legs. These types of injections may be used to help relieve leg or arm pain resulting from damage to or pressure on a large peripheral nerve.

Medications

The most common types of medication used in peripheral joint and nerve injections are local anesthetics and steroid medications. The drugs may be given separately or combined into one shot:

- **Local anesthetic.** A local anesthetic is used to temporarily numb a painful area. It works by interfering with, or blocking, pain pathways to the brain. The result is less pain in that area. You may also experience

Greater occipital nerve

Needle

Occipital injection

An occipital injection is performed at the base of the skull, blocking transmission of signals from the occipital nerve. The occipital nerves originate in the upper (cervical) spine.

reduced feeling at the location of the injection because the nerves have been numbed.

- **Steroid.** Long-acting injected steroid medications help decrease pain by reducing inflammation in joints and around nerves. Steroids may be injected into one or several affected areas of your body, such as the shoulder, elbow, hip or knee. In the short term, corticosteroids can make you feel dramatically better and they may provide pain relief for two to three months. But when used for many months or years, they may cause serious side effects, such as weakened cartilage and ligaments, easy bruising, thinning of bones, cataracts, weight gain, a

Injections of hyaluronic acid in the knee joint

The past number of years, a compound called hyaluronic acid — more commonly known by the brand names Synvisc and Hyalgan — has been injected into knee joints to help treat osteoarthritis of the knee.

Hyaluronic acid is a lubricating substance found in normal joint fluid. In people with osteoarthritis, hyaluronic acid often thins out and there isn't enough of the acid to provide adequate protection to the joint. In an attempt to improve lubrication and joint mobility, a compound containing hyaluronic acid is injected into the knee joint in a series of shots.

There's some controversy as to whether these injections are effective. Recent studies and reviews suggest that the injections aren't very effective. They may help some people initially, but the benefits generally don't last beyond six months. There's also no evidence they slow progression of the disease.

round face, diabetes, high blood pressure, and a decreased ability to heal wounds and fight infections.

Soft tissue injections

When a specific part of your body — such as a muscle or bursa — is inflamed and painful, an injection may be given directly into the surrounding soft tissue. There are two main types of soft tissue injections.

Trigger point injections. Trigger points are areas where your muscles and surrounding connective tissue are sensitive to touch. Trigger points are generally located in the upper and lower back muscles, but may occur elsewhere. Trigger point injections are used when muscles are overly sensitive and are a source of pain. Depending on the medication used, trigger point injections may help reduce pain in a muscle, reduce inflammation or relax an overly sensitive muscle.

Bursa injections. Bursae are tiny, fluid-filled sacs that lubricate and cushion pressure points between your bones and the tendons and muscles near your joints. You have more than 150 bursae in your body, which help you move without pain. When bursae become

Trigger points
The areas highlighted in green are some common trigger points. Medication may be injected in these areas to relieve pain in overly sensitive muscles.

Trochanteric bursa

Needle

Bursa injection
A local anesthetic and steroid medication are injected into a bursa to reduce the pain and inflammation of bursitis.

inflamed (bursitis), movement of or pressure on the affected joint becomes painful. Bursitis most often affects the shoulder, elbow or hip areas.

Medication

Medications used in soft tissue injections include:

- **Local anesthetic.** A local anesthetic is used to provide immediate pain relief. Often an anesthetic is given in conjunction with a steroid medication, but sometimes an anesthetic may be given alone.

- **Steroid.** A corticosteroid medication is injected into soft tissue to help reduce inflammation. It may take three to four days before the medication starts working. Reducing inflammation and pain allows for increased movement in the affected area. Effects may last from a few weeks to several months.

- **Botox.** A type of toxin known as botulinum toxin is injected into one or more muscles causing pain. The toxin causes temporary paralysis of these muscles. Botox injections may be used if you have a condition caused by cramping muscles (dystonia), certain types of headaches

or other disorders involving chronic muscle spasm. The amount of toxin used is very small. Its effects generally last about three months. Repeat injections are often needed.

Spinal injections

Spinal injections are used in situations in which chronic pain is thought to be associated with a spinal joint or nerve that's been damaged or is irritated or inflamed. A local anesthetic may be injected to numb the pain, a steroid medication given to reduce inflammation, or a combination of both.

An injection directly into the spinal fluid is called an intrathecal (in-truh-THEE-kul) injection. This type of injection is often used during surgery on the abdomen or lower extremities. If the injection isn't into the spinal fluid, it's called an epidural injection. Epidurals are often used to relieve the pain of childbirth and sometimes are given to relieve some types of back pain, such as sciatica.

In addition to treating pain, spinal injections can help diagnose the cause of pain. If medication placed in a certain location relieves the pain, doctors are able to focus on the pain source.

Epidural injection

An epidural injection is performed under X-ray guidance. A needle is positioned in the epidural space in the spinal column, and medications are injected to relieve the pain.

Spinal injections are performed with the guidance of fluoroscopy, an X-ray imaging procedure that allows the doctor or imaging specialist to view the spinal column as the needle containing the medication is inserted. For this procedure, you may be asked to lie facedown on the examining table or on your side.

There are several types of spinal injections. Some of the more common injections include:

- **Epidural.** Epidural injections are the most common. The needle is inserted between the back bones into the epidural space that sur-

rounds the spinal cord and spinal nerves. Epidural injections may be given in the neck (cervical), mid-back (thoracic) and low back (lumbar). The medication coats nerves in the location where it's injected, relieving pain.

- **Transforaminal epidural.** In these injections, the needle containing medication is inserted into the epidural space through the opening of an exiting nerve root. This technique allows the medication to be placed closer to a nerve root responsible for the pain than does the standard epidural approach.

- **Selective nerve root.** In this type of injection, medication is placed around the nerve root after it leaves the spine. This type of injection is used mostly to diagnose a painful condition. It can help determine which nerve root is the predominant source of pain.

- **Facet joint.** In this procedure, medication is injected into one or more facet joints — small, stabilizing joints located between and behind the spine's vertebrae. The medication, typically a steroid, reduces inflammation and swelling of tissue within the joint that's causing pain.

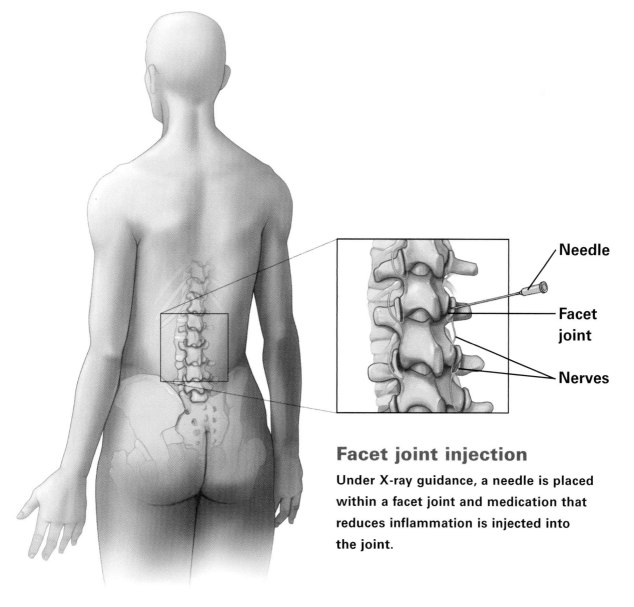

Needle

Facet joint

Nerves

Facet joint injection

Under X-ray guidance, a needle is placed within a facet joint and medication that reduces inflammation is injected into the joint.

- **Sympathetic block.** With this type of injection, medication is inserted into nerve tissue that's part of the sympathetic nervous system. The sympathetic nerves are located in the back and neck on either side of the spine. Sympathetic blocks help reduce pain and swelling, as well as color and sweating changes in the legs and feet. The injections are used to treat conditions such as complex regional pain syndrome.

- **Celiac plexus block.** A local anesthetic is injected into a group of nerves that serve the body's abdominal organs (celiac plexus nerves). This type of block is performed most often to treat chronic upper abdominal pain and pain from pancreatic cancer.

- **Sacroiliac joint.** These types of injections are given in the sacroiliac joint in the buttock region. They're used to treat a type of low back-buttock pain.

- **Piriformis muscle.** This type of injection may be used in people experiencing impingement of the sciatic nerve as the nerve passes through the piriformis muscle, a muscle located behind the hip joint. Medication is injected into the muscle in an attempt to relieve the pain.

- **Discogram.** This procedure is used to determine which disk or disks in your back are causing pain. A solution is injected into one or more disks in an attempt to re-create the pain by increasing pressure in the disk.

Piriformis muscle

Sacroilliac joint

Sacroiliac and piriformis injections

In these procedures, medication is injected into the sacroiliac joint or piriformis muscle to relieve low back or leg pain.

- **Radiofrequency ablation.** For this procedure, a needle used in conjunction with nerve stimulation is placed near a painful nerve. Heat produced by radio waves (high-frequency energy) runs through the needle to the nerve, heats up nerve tissue and disrupts pain signals coming from the tissue. The disruption blocks nerve signals to the brain. The procedure isn't a permanent treatment. The nerves often grow back, and the procedure may need to be repeated.

Nerve stimulators

Nerve stimulators are electronic devices that produce electrical signals to stimulate certain nerves, with the goal of reducing pain. They include transcutaneous electrical nerve stimulators (TENS), spinal cord stimulators and peripheral nerve stimulators.

TENS

For this type of nerve stimulation, electrodes are placed on your skin near the painful area. The electrodes are then attached to a small, portable, battery-powered unit. The unit generates low-level, painless electric impulses that pass through your skin to underlying nerve fibers to modify your pain perception. You adjust settings on the TENS unit as needed to control the level of electric impulse.

Exactly how TENS works isn't known. It may trigger the release of endorphins — chemicals in your body that have painkilling effects similar to the drug morphine. TENS treatment may also block nerve pathways that carry pain messages.

TENS generally works best for mild pain, and not all people who use the device benefit from it. Most often, TENS is combined with exercise and other pain treatments.

A similar treatment called percutaneous electrical nerve stimulation (PENS) is used in combination with acupuncture. Instead of transmitting the current through electrodes placed on top of your skin, PENS uses thin needles that penetrate your skin to just below its surface. Most people feel some sensation, but not pain, when the needles are inserted. Unlike TENS, percutaneous electrical nerve stimulation must be performed by a trained practitioner and cannot be used at home or at work.

Spinal cord and peripheral nerve stimulators

Spinal cord and peripheral nerve stimulators may be a treatment option for people who suffer from certain types of chronic pain conditions. These electronic devices aren't a cure for the pain. Rather, their objective is to reduce the pain to a more manageable level.

Spinal cord and peripheral nerve stimulators are most often used when traditional treatments for pain, such as medication or surgery, are ineffective, not feasible or they cause unwanted side effects.

During a short surgical procedure, a thin wire called a lead is placed in the space that surrounds the spinal cord and spinal nerves (epidural space) or alongside a large peripheral nerve — depending on the type and source of your pain. An electrical generator also is inserted under the skin. The lead is connected to the generator, and when the generator's power is turned on, electrical power is sent

through the lead to an electrode — in the form a needle — attached at the other end. The electrode stimulates nerve fibers at the location where you're experiencing pain. The hope is that the stimulation will alter the pain messages and replace them with more pleasant sensations (paresthesia). These sensations differ, but people often describe them as a tingling feeling.

There are different types of neurostimulation, and the type that's right for you depends on many factors, including the cause of your pain or neurological disorder, as well as its type and location. Recent improvements to spinal cord stimulators include rechargeable batteries. An external device held over the implanted unit recharges the battery, reducing the number of surgeries needed to replace worn-out batteries.

If you're a candidate for spinal cord or peripheral nerve stimulation, you'll likely undergo a stimulation trial to find out how well you respond to the therapy before you commit to surgery to fully implant the system. For some people the sensation emitted by the stimulator isn't pleasant nor does it relieve the pain.

Electrode or catheter

Drug infusion device or electrical generator placed beneath the skin

With a nerve stimulator, an electrode is placed in the epidural space within the spinal canal.

With a pain pump, medication is administered through a catheter to the intrathecal space in the spinal canal.

Nerve stimulators and pain pumps

Each of these procedures is performed under X-ray guidance. With both procedures, a needle is inserted into the correct location. In the case of a nerve stimulator, an electrode is then positioned in the epidural space and the needle is removed. With a pain pump, the needle is inserted into the intrathecal space and is removed once a catheter that administers the medication is positioned correctly.

Medication pumps

Commonly referred to as medication pumps or pain pumps, the technical term for these devices is *intrathecal drug delivery systems.* They deliver pain medication directly to the fluid that surrounds the spinal cord (cerebrospinal fluid).

Medication pumps are most often used to treat cancer pain and chronic pain that doesn't respond to other types of treatment. This may include pain resulting from nerve damage or illness and pain associated with muscle spasm resulting from injury to the spinal cord.

A medication pump consists of a small flexible catheter that's placed in the spinal fluid. The catheter is connected to a drug infusion pump that's implanted into your lower abdomen. The medication is placed into the pump via a small covered opening (port) in the top of the pump.

A computerized program tells the pump how much of the medication you are to receive, dispensing the drug at a set rate. The medication may be an opioid (narcotic) or a local anesthetic, muscle relaxant or other medication. The muscle relaxant baclofen (Lioresal) or the new analgesic medication ziconotide (Prialt) may be used. Ziconotide was developed specifically for use in medication pumps.

This method of drug delivery may reduce your pain and cause fewer side effects than oral pain medications. This is because less medication may be needed when the medication is delivered directly to pain receptors in the spinal cord.

Similar to a spinal cord stimulator, your doctor will likely recommend that you first undergo a screening trial before the device is permanently implanted to see if the treatment will help you.

You may have to restrict some activities while using a medication pump. That's because the pain medication being dispensed may produce numbness, which can reduce your ability to sense pressure and temperature changes, in addition to pain. The numbness often decreases with time, but it may not go away entirely. Another drawback of these devices is that they're expensive.

Choosing the right treatment

The procedures and technologies described in this chapter offer a variety of treatment options. Keep in mind that these options don't exclude one another. For instance, someone with chronic pain may receive physical therapy as well as use a spinal cord stimulator.

Selecting a technology that's best for you involves consideration of several factors. Be sure to discuss the issues below — as well as any other questions you have — with your doctor.

Your expectations. Stimulators and medication pumps represent the latest in pain management technology. However, no technology offers total pain relief. Technology can lessen your discomfort, but you'll probably continue to feel some pain. A reasonable goal is to reduce your pain by 50 percent.

Your treatment history. Before prescribing devices such as implantable stimulators and pumps, your doctor may first try a variety of other treatments, such as oral medication, physical therapy, exercise and counseling.

Stimulators and pumps are generally recommended only after you've tried less invasive and less expensive options. Knowing how you've responded to pain treatments in the past can help predict how well a new technology may work for you.

Your medical evaluation. In addition to standard tests, such as checking your blood pressure and heart rate, your doctor may require that you have a psychological evaluation. A psychological evaluation recognizes that your mind and body are connected. The success of any medical treatment may depend in part on your feelings about the treatment as well as how you cope with pain on a day-to-day basis.

Medical risks and side effects. Surgery is needed to implant any device in your body, and any surgery carries some risk. In addition, pain medications have side effects — a factor to consider with injections or any device that delivers medication.

Your range of pain. When chronic pain is localized in a particular area of your body, injections or peripheral nerve stimulation may be the best option. For pain that spreads over a larger region of your body, a spinal cord stimulator or medication pump might be more useful. But again, no technology offers total pain relief.

Your comfort level. Like any piece of technology, pumps and stimulators require general maintenance and troubleshooting. Most spinal cord stimulators in use today have a rechargeable battery that you need to recharge. Pump batteries aren't rechargeable and must be changed from time to time. Pumps must also be refilled with medication. Be sure that you fully understand all that's involved in using a pump or stimulator.

Where you live and travel. If your medication pump runs out of medication or malfunctions, you may experience withdrawal symptoms, changes in blood pressure or other complications. During such a situation, you'll need to get to a doctor. This may be a factor in determining the best treatment for you.

Insurance coverage. Most medical insurers will cover the cost of pain relief technology, but you'll need to work with your doctor and insurance company in order to satisfy requirements for coverage.

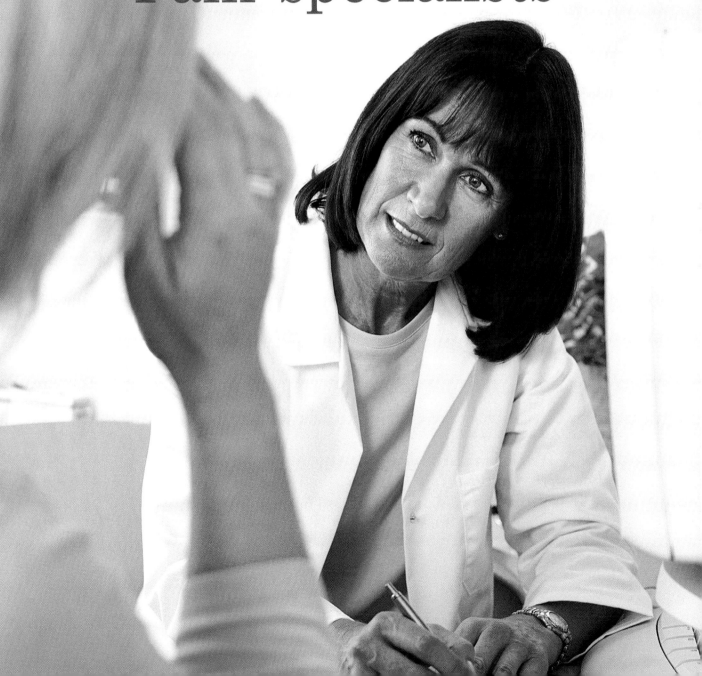

Chapter 8

Pain specialists

Major life changes sometimes require personal guidance. Learning how to manage chronic pain is one instance where one-on-one help may make a difference. If you feel that you might benefit from more individualized care, you may want to see an individual who specializes in pain medicine. Or, perhaps, your primary care doctor has recommended that you see a pain specialist.

Pain specialists, or pain medicine doctors, can help diagnose the cause of your pain — provided a cause can be found — as well as develop a plan for treating the pain. However, you need to be careful. Not all doctors who claim to be pain specialists have received extensive training. Make sure you see a doctor who's certified in pain medicine.

What's a pain specialist?

Pain specialists are doctors who work closely with your primary care physician to assess the cause of your pain and determine appropriate treatment. Doctors who have received extensive training in the treatment of pain often are board certified in the field of pain medicine. The types of doctors who most frequently specialize in pain management, and who are eligible for pain medicine certification, include the following:

- **Anesthesiologists.** These are doctors who are trained to relieve pain. In addition to preventing pain during and after surgery, anesthesiologists may also have specialty training in the treatment of chronic pain.
- **Neurologists.** Neurologists are doctors who diagnose and treat diseases of the nervous system.
- **Physiatrists.** Physiatrists are doctors who are trained in the field of physical medicine and rehabilitation (PM&R), a branch of medicine that deals with treatment and prevention of disease by physical means, including exercise, manipulation and massage.
- **Psychiatrists.** Psychiatry is the branch of medicine devoted to the diagnosis and treatment of mental health disorders.

In addition to psychiatrists, some psychologists also specialize in the treatment of chronic pain. Because psychologists are not medical doctors, they aren't eligible for pain medicine certification. However, psychologists may receive accreditation from the American Board of Professional Psychology in Health.

What's a pain clinic?

A pain clinic is the name often given to a medical facility that specializes in the treatment of chronic pain. Some facilities use the term *center* instead of *clinic*. A pain clinic, or center, may specialize in the treatment of a specific type of pain, such as headache or back pain, or it may treat an array of painful conditions.

Some pain clinics are associated with a medical institution, such as a pain clinic located within a hospital or medical center. Other pain clinics are stand-alone facilities that are run by one or more individual doctors.

Another way in which pain clinics differ is that some focus on only one type of pain treatment — for instance, the use of medication to relieve pain, either in the form of pills or injections. This compares with more broad-based pain clinics, which rely on a variety of treatments — from psychological counseling to physical therapy to acupuncture — to help manage pain.

Similar to seeing your primary care doctor, a pain specialist located at a pain clinic will likely perform a thorough medical history and physical exam. Additional diagnostic tests may also be performed. These tests may include X-rays or diagnostic nerve blocks. If the cause of your pain is found, the next step is often developing a treatment plan to address the pain source. If a cause can't be found, a pain specialist will work with you on different ways to control the pain to keep it at a manageable level.

Working as a team

Doctors who specialize in the treatment of chronic pain often don't work alone. This is especially true for broad-based pain clinics that treat a variety of conditions and that use a multifaceted approach to managing pain. In this type of setting, a pain specialist may lead or be part of a team that may include some or all of the following:

Other doctors. In addition to specialists in pain medicine, the facility may also include other doctors who treat specific forms of pain, including anesthesiologists, neurologists, psychiatrists, or physical medicine and rehabilitation physicians (physiatrists).

Psychologists. Psychologists teach strategies to cope with pain and improve daily functioning. They also address the behavioral and emotional issues that can accompany chronic pain, such as depression and fear, and they help identify issues that may be contributing to the pain, such as strained family relations or stress at work.

Nurses. Nurses often oversee medication use or medication withdrawal. They may monitor your progress and act as a case manager, serving as your advocate and acting as an intermediary to other professionals on the team.

Physical and occupational therapists. The role of therapists is to help rebuild your strength and endurance and to instill confidence in your ability to function in everyday life. Physical therapists do this through individualized instruction in a complete exercise and fitness program. Occupational

therapists, meanwhile, focus on increasing your competency in specific day-to-day tasks.

Others. Additional professionals may include a registered dietitian, a social worker and a vocational counselor.

What to look for

Because pain clinics and centers vary in their qualifications and specialties, consider these factors when evaluating your options:

- **What are the goals of the program?** Is the program focused strictly on relieving your pain? Or does it include services to help determine the cause of your pain or personal problems that may be associated with your pain?
- **What methods does the program advocate?** Be cautious of programs that advocate long-term use of potentially addictive drugs, such as narcotics, or that routinely include surgery or rely on unproven alternative therapies.
- **Are staff members friendly and willing to listen?** It's important that you feel comfortable with those around you. Staff should be

interested in you and willing to take time to listen.

- **Is your doctor willing to answer questions?** Questions may include: Do you have experience in treating my kind of pain? How long have you been practicing? Are you certified in pain management?

- **Is the program accredited or certified?** Pain centers or clinics don't have to be accredited or certified to operate. However, certification helps ensure that the program meets basic requirements.

- **Does it have a good success rate?** Ask what the long-term success rate of the program is. Keep in mind that no clinic or center can offer a 100 percent success rate.

- **Does it include follow-up services?** If you need additional care once you've completed your treatment, there should be a phone number to call or person to contact.

- **How much does it cost?** Know approximately what the treatment will cost before you start. Check with your insurance company to see what expenses are covered. Some insurance companies cover treatment provided by pain programs, while others don't.

Chapter 9

Pain rehabilitation centers

With chronic pain, there often isn't an effective treatment that can make the pain go away. This can be a hard pill to swallow, especially if you've spent a lot of time and money hoping to relieve your pain. But it doesn't mean that all is lost. While you may not be able to make the pain disappear, you can learn how to cope with it.

With the right tools and techniques, it's possible to reduce your pain and improve your quality of life. Your doctor or a pain specialist may offer advice on how to manage your pain. You might also consider visiting a pain rehabilitation center, provided you live in a location with such a facility nearby, or you're willing to travel to a medical

center that offers such a program. Pain rehabilitation programs are designed to reverse the downward course that can occur with chronic pain — helping you learn how to control your pain so that you can enjoy life, instead of letting your pain control you.

Rehabilitation programs

Pain rehabilitation programs support the belief that chronic pain affects many aspects of your life and, therefore, requires a broad treatment approach. These programs explore various ways

Is a pain rehabilitation program right for me?

Pain rehabilitation is a challenging process that requires a serious commitment. Ask yourself these questions to assess your readiness:

- Is my life controlled by pain?
- Are my doctors telling me they can do nothing further to relieve my pain?
- Am I concerned about the long-term effects of taking pain medications?
- Is my family's well-being affected by my pain?
- Is my recovery from injury or illness taking much longer than my doctors or I expected?
- Am I not able to commit to events with family or friends because of worry about controlling my pain?

to help you control your pain. In addition, they help you identify factors that may contribute to your pain. The programs are generally intended for people who have experienced a significant decline in their daily functioning and quality of life, as a result of their pain.

In most pain rehabilitation programs, pain specialists integrate behavioral and lifestyle changes with physical and occupational therapy and, occasionally, selective use of medications or injections. Depending on the location or cause of your pain, other therapies, such as relaxation techniques, stress management and complementary medicine, also may be incorporated into your treatment plan.

Most pain rehabilitation programs are located within large academic centers, and they include a large staff of doctors, nurses, psychologists, physical and occupational therapists and other health professionals. The primary goal of these programs, which have been in existence for more than 30 years, is to restore physical functioning and improve the quality of life for people with unrelieved pain.

Common goals of most pain rehabilitation programs include:

- Return to regular daily activities
- Elimination or reduction of pain medications that are of little or no benefit or cause adverse side effects
- Increased physical strength, stamina and flexibility
- Use of stress management and relaxation techniques
- Return to employment (if applicable)
- Resumption of leisure and recreational activities
- Improved relations with family, friends and co-workers
- Reduced reliance on health care professionals

What to expect

Not all pain rehabilitation programs operate in exactly the same way, but their approach is often quite similar.

Once you've been admitted into the program, you'll likely receive a thorough evaluation. This may include having staff review your physical and psychological condition, use of medication, work situation and relationships with family and friends. In addition to helping staff devise a treatment plan, the evaluation is helpful in setting goals that address your specific needs. Your goals might include getting off your medication, becoming more physically active, learning to relax or returning to work.

In some rehabilitation programs, the therapy and attention you receive are intensive. You spend most of the day at the center for two to four weeks. During this time, you work with physical and occupational therapists and spend time in group sessions. You also meet regularly with your case manager to discuss your progress, as well as areas that remain difficult for you. With other rehabilitation programs, the schedule is less intensive. You meet for just a few hours a week over several weeks.

Similar to pain clinics and centers, before enrolling in a pain rehabilitation program, make sure it's a reputable program and that it's a good fit for

Are pain rehabilitation programs effective?

Mayo Clinic's Comprehensive Pain Rehabilitation Center, founded in 1974, was one of the first pain rehabilitation centers in the United States. It's now one of the largest in the nation. The center offers an intensive three-week program that serves approximately 400 people annually.

As part of its mission to help people with chronic pain improve their quality of life, the center conducts ongoing research as to the effectiveness of the program. Treatment outcomes from individuals who have completed Mayo's program, shown below, are likely comparable to those at other reputable pain rehabilitation centers across the country. Participants were able to retain these benefits for at least six months.

Patient satisfaction. The majority of participants — 91 percent — "strongly agreed" or "agreed" that the pain rehabilitation center was beneficial in helping them learn how to live well in spite of chronic pain.

Medication. Upon completion of the program, 4 percent of participants were still taking opioid (narcotic) medications, compared with 45 percent at admission. Use of nonsteroidal anti-inflammatory drugs (NSAIDs) and muscle relaxants also decreased.

Depression. Scores on the Center for Epidemiological Studies Depression Scale (CES-D) showed a 79 percent reduction from admission to discharge among people experiencing depressive symptoms.

Physical therapy. Seventy-five percent of people completing the program had at least a 50 percent gain in their aerobic activity level. More than 20 percent of participants experienced a gain of 75 percent or more in their level of aerobic activity.

Pain severity. In rehabilitation, pain reduction is not a program goal, and there are no medical or surgical procedures to specifically reduce pain. However, because participants learn coping strategies for managing pain while improving the quality of their life, 73 percent of those completing the program report a reduction in the severity of their pain.

Confidence level. Eighty-four percent of participants note increased feelings of control over pain and life events.

you. It's also important that your family be involved in your care. Look for a program that provides educational sessions for family members.

To find a reputable pain program that fits your needs, talk with your doctor. Organizations that may provide references include the American Pain Society and the American Academy of Pain Medicine (see page 240).

Chapter 10

Complementary and alternative medicine

In your quest to find relief from your pain, chances are you've tried or considered some form of complementary or alternative medicine. Maybe you've had a massage, practiced meditation or yoga, or thought about acupuncture or herbal medicines.

And you probably have a lot of questions. Do these methods really work? Are they safe? Exactly what is complementary and alternative medicine? This chapter helps answer these questions.

The National Center for Complementary and Alternative Medicine (NCCAM), a division of the National Institutes of Health, defines complementary medicine as unconventional treatments used in addition to treatments by your doctor. An example would be practicing meditation in addition to taking prescription drugs to manage anxiety.

In contrast, alternative medicine includes treatments used in place of traditional medicine. This might include seeing a homeopath or natur-opath instead of your regular doctor.

Among the general public, however, this distinction isn't as clear. Many people use the term *alternative medicine* as a catchall phrase to refer to both — those therapies used in addition to conventional care and those used in place of it.

Integrative medicine, meanwhile, is a fairly new term that describes a grow-ing movement taking place in many health care institutions — integrating complementary and alternative thera-pies with conventional medicine. The goal of integrative medicine is to treat the whole person — mind, body and spirit — not just the disease. This is done by combining the best of today's high-tech medicine with the best of nontraditional practices — practices that have some high-quality evidence to support their use.

Complementary and alternative thera-pies aren't new. Some have been prac-ticed for thousands of years. But their use has become more popular as peo-ple seek greater control of their own health. Two of the most common con-ditions for which people use comple-mentary and alternative medicine are

anxiety and pain. Studies sponsored by NCCAM have shown that certain ther-apies, such as biofeedback, meditation and relaxed breathing, can be useful in treating chronic pain. For others, the evidence isn't as supportive.

5 smart strategies

Complementary and alternative medicine can play a role in better health. But it's important to remember that there are some important differ-ences between conventional medicine and complementary and alternative therapies and practices.

If you decide to use complementary and alternative treatments, protecting your health — and your wallet — requires you to do two things. First, find out how various treatments work and what benefits they may provide. Second, take responsibility for your own well-being. Before selecting a spe-cific treatment, do your homework.

1. **Gather information about the treatment.** The Internet offers an ideal way to keep up with the latest

on complementary and alternative treatments — a fast-changing field. If you don't have Internet access at home or work, then contact your local library to see whether it offers Web access to the public.

2. **Find and evaluate treatment providers.** After gathering information about a treatment, look for a qualified practitioner. Whenever possible, talk to people who've received the treatment you're considering and ask about their experience with specific treatment providers. Before you receive a treatment, call the provider and schedule an informational appointment to learn more about the procedure or therapy. With any treatment

Sounds too good to be true? Maybe it is.

The Food and Drug Administration and the National Council Against Health Fraud recommend that you watch for the following claims or practices to protect yourself against potentially fraudulent treatments:

- Promotional materials include words such as *breakthrough, magical* or *new discovery*. If the product were in fact a cure, it would be widely reported in the media and your doctor would prescribe it.
- Promotional materials include pseudomedical jargon such as *detoxify, purify* or *energize.* Such claims are difficult to measure.
- The manufacturer claims that the product can treat a wide range of diseases and conditions. No single product can do this.
- The product is supposedly backed by scientific studies, but references aren't provided, are limited or are out-of-date.
- The product's promotional materials mention no negative side effects, only benefits.
- The manufacturer accuses the government or medical profession of suppressing important information about the product's benefits.

you consider, determine if the benefits outweigh the risks.

3. **Consider treatment costs.** Many complementary and alternative approaches aren't covered by health insurance. Find out exactly how much the treatment will cost you and get the total amount in writing before you start treatment.

4. **Check your attitude.** When it comes to complementary and alternative medicine, steer a middle course between uncritical acceptance and outright rejection. Learn to be open-minded and skeptical at the same time. Keep your mind open to different treatment options but evaluate them carefully.

5. **Opt for a combined approach.** Research indicates that the best use of unconventional medicine is to complement rather than replace traditional medical care. Use complementary and alternative therapies in conjunction with the treatment being prescribed by your doctor. While complementary and alternative therapies can help you maintain good health and relieve some symptoms, it's important that you continue to rely on conventional medicine to diagnose a problem and treat your condition. Make sure to tell your health care team about all of the treatments you're using — both conventional and unconventional.

Also remember that there's no substitute for a healthy lifestyle. Nutrition, exercise, stress management and adequate rest are key to improved health and relief of pain.

Herbs and other supplements

As anyone who's walked through a health food store can attest, the profusion of herbal remedies and other dietary supplements is almost overwhelming. Following are some products heavily marketed for pain relief — especially arthritic pain.

Devil's claw

The herb devil's claw originates from the Kalahari Desert region of southern Africa. It's used to relieve pain and inflammation in joints and to treat headache and back pain. The manner

Evaluating herbal remedies

Unlike medications you receive from your doctor, dietary and herbal products aren't regulated by the Food and Drug Administration (FDA) for effectiveness. Regulations regarding the safety of these products also are different.

With prescription drugs, the manufacturer must prove that the benefits of the drug outweigh any safety concerns before the drug is approved for sale. Dietary and herbal supplements, however, are assumed to be safe until proved otherwise. Only when a supplement is found unsafe is it removed from the market. Because these products don't follow the same safety procedures, they can contain toxic substances that may not be listed on the label. In addition, the amount of active ingredient may vary greatly between different brands.

You might consider herbal products to be natural and, therefore, harmless. However, they can have active chemicals that may not safely mix with other medications you're taking. The best advice is to talk with your doctor before taking any dietary supplement or herbal product.

in which it works is unknown. Research suggests devil's claw may be effective for short-term treatment of osteoarthritic pain, and it may also help alleviate low back pain. But the studies have been small, and more information is needed before any type of recommendations can be made regarding use of this herb for pain relief.

Glucosamine and chondroitin

Glucosamine and chondroitin are natural compounds found in cartilage — the tough tissue that cushions joints. They're used to treat osteoarthritis, a painful condition caused by the inflammation, breakdown and loss of cartilage. Glucosamine supplements are made from the skeletons of shellfish (chitin). Chondroitin supplements are made from cow and shark cartilage, as well as from other sources.

Glucosamine and chondroitin have become an extremely popular treatment for osteoarthritis. They appear to be safe and produce fewer adverse side effects than do medications such as nonsteroidal anti-inflammatory drugs (NSAIDs). The question is, are they effective at treating arthritis? While

many older studies gave very promising results, the results of a large study sponsored by the National Institutes of Health were mostly negative. The only individuals who appeared to receive some benefit were those with very severe symptoms.

However, while the studies may be conflicting, side effects from the supplements are few and far between. So far, no other treatments have shown promise at increasing cartilage. It's possible — though certainly not guaranteed — glucosamine and chondroitin may help.

SAM-e

S-adenosylmethionine (SAM-e) is a compound that occurs naturally in the human body. Among other functions, it helps produce and regulate hormones and maintain cell membranes. Trials indicate that SAM-e can relieve pain from osteoarthritis as effectively as NSAIDs, with fewer side effects.

But the long-term benefits and risks of SAM-e are still unknown. As with any supplement, it's best to consult your doctor before trying SAM-e. One drawback of SAM-e is that it can interact with antidepressant medications.

Hands-on therapies

This group includes some of the most commonly used complementary treatments. Hands-on therapies are often used to treat musculoskeletal conditions such as back pain, headache and arthritis.

Aromatherapy

This ancient form of healing involves the use of essential oils that are derived from plant extracts and resins and used to promote both health and healing. Practitioners believe these oils can help treat various symptoms and conditions — including pain — when massaged into your skin or inhaled.

There are about 150 different essential oils used in aromatherapy. The oils are categorized according to their effects on the mind and body and on specific diseases. More study is needed to determine whether these oils provide any health benefit, and for which conditions they may be the most beneficial. Aromatherapy is often used in conjunction with massage therapy (see page 131).

Chiropractic

Chiropractic therapy is perhaps the most common complementary therapy in the United States. Chiropractic treatment is based on the concept that restricted movement in the spine may lead to pain and reduced function. Spinal adjustment (manipulation) is one form of therapy chiropractors use to treat restricted spinal mobility. The goal is to restore spinal movement and, as a result, improve function and decrease back pain.

Studies have found spinal manipulation to be an effective treatment for uncomplicated low back pain, especially if the pain has been present less than four weeks. Studies also suggest spinal manipulation may be effective for headache and other spine-related conditions, such as neck pain. There's no evidence, though, to support the belief that spinal manipulation can cure whatever ails you.

As with any medical specialist, select a chiropractor who's willing to work with the other members of your health care team. Make sure you're comfortable with the recommendations, including how many sessions you'll need. Be questionable of chiropractors who ask to extend your treatment indefinitely.

When limited to the low back, chiropractic treatment has few risks. However, manipulation of the neck has been associated with injury to blood vessels supplying the brain. Rarely, neck manipulation may cause a stroke.

Massage

Massage therapy involves the use of different manipulative techniques to move your body's muscles and soft tissues. Massage therapists primarily use their hands to manipulate muscles and tissues, but sometimes they may use their forearms, elbows or feet.

Massage therapy is based on the belief that when muscles are overworked, waste products can accumulate in the muscle, causing soreness and stiffness. The aim of massage therapy is to improve circulation in the muscle, increasing the flow of nutrients and oxygen and eliminating waste products. In addition, massage induces the body's relaxation response, another route to healing and improved health.

Massage therapists claim that their treatment can help relieve stress and anxiety, relax your muscles, help relieve headaches, lower blood pressure, improve range of motion in your joints, and increase production of your body's natural painkillers.

A growing body of literature is beginning to validate many of the benefits of massage therapy. Studies suggest it can help decrease headache pain and pain associated with fibromyalgia. It may also help relieve back pain. Although massage is generally safe, avoid it if you have open sores, acute inflammation or circulatory problems. A massage should feel good. If it doesn't, speak up.

Movement therapies

Several nontraditional therapies, such as the Feldenkrais and Trager methods, center around the philosophy that, over time, people start moving and holding their bodies in dysfunctional ways. Weaker muscles end up doing the work of stronger muscles, causing stress and tension.

With these therapies, an instructor takes you through a series of specific movements designed to teach you to use your muscles and joints more comfortably and efficiently. The movements are also designed to help you find greater ease with your body.

Practitioners claim these therapies can help control pain and promote an overall sense of well-being. Although they appear to be safe, their benefits aren't scientifically supported.

Prolotherapy

Prolotherapy — also known as sclerotherapy or proliferant therapy — is a procedure done by a trained professional that involves injecting painful ligaments and tendons with sterile solutions containing dextrose, a specific type of sugar. The solutions are intended to stimulate the production of connective tissue. Proponents of prolotherapy believe that the treatments help restore strength and stability to ligaments and joints, which in turn helps relieve pain. Prolotherapy has been used to treat a number of painful musculoskeletal conditions, such as osteoarthritis and chronic back pain.

Studies of prolotherapy have produced conflicting evidence regarding its effectiveness in treating chronic pain. Some have suggested a possible benefit, while others have indicated none. At this point, more research is needed to determine what role, if any, prolotherapy may play in the treatment of chronic pain.

Rolfing

This form of hands-on therapy uses deep massage to align your body so that all of its components are positioned correctly. The theory behind Rolfing is that injury or stress causes tissues to adhere in unhealthy ways, interfering with your body's natural movement and producing symptoms such as pain. To restore natural alignment, a therapist applies deep pressure to stretch the tissues and help reposition muscles and joints.

There are no scientific studies to support Rolfing's benefits. Its deep massage may help reduce stress and tension. However, some people find the procedure painful, and it may worsen chronic pain.

Energy therapies

Energy therapies are based on the belief that the body contains natural energy fields and that good health results when this energy can flow freely without interruption.

Acupressure and acupuncture

These therapies stem from the Chinese belief that within the human body there are multiple invisible pathways, called meridians. Through these pathways flows qi (pronounced chee), the Chinese word for "life force" or "life energy." When the flow of qi is obstructed, illness or pain results.

During acupressure, a practitioner applies pressure with his or her fingers to specific points on your body in an attempt to restore the free flow of qi and relieve symptoms such as pain and stress. People who feel they're helped by the procedure find the therapy to be relaxing and comforting. However, more research is needed to document the effectiveness of this treatment.

During a typical acupuncture session, an acupuncturist inserts anywhere from one to 20 hair-thin needles into your skin for 10 to 30 minutes. The acupuncturist may also manipulate the needles or apply electrical stimulation or heat to the needles.

Acupuncture is one of the most studied nontraditional medical practices, and it's gaining acceptance within modern medicine for treatment of certain conditions.

A number of studies have shown that acupuncture is effective in treating postoperative dental pain, pain related to endoscopic procedures, low back pain related to pregnancy and some forms of chronic pain, including fibromyalgic pain. Acupuncture has also been effective in reducing pain related to tennis elbow, but it's had mixed results when used to treat osteoarthritis of the knee, hip and back. Some studies suggest it may provide considerable pain relief, while other studies show no benefit.

Adverse side effects from acupuncture are rare, but they can occur. Make sure your acupuncturist is trained and certified or licensed and follows good hygiene practices, including use of disposable needles.

Magnet therapy

Most claims regarding the healing power of magnets are from manufacturers of products that contain magnets. These products include arm and leg wraps, belts, mattress pads and shoe inserts. Manufacturers often claim the products can relieve various health problems, including chronic pain, by stimulating your body's natural electrical field.

To date, there's no scientific evidence that magnets used in this manner provide any health benefits. And some experts believe inappropriate use of magnets could possibly lead to health problems.

A few medical researchers are exploring the use of different, more powerful magnets — not the common refrigerator magnets — as a therapy for some forms of chronic pain. More study is needed before any conclusions can be drawn.

Mind-body therapies

A simple definition of mind-body medicine reads like this: "positively influencing the mind to improve the health of the individual." The belief that mind and body are intricately connected goes back centuries. Mind-body practices have two core components. The first is to restore the mind to a state of peaceful neutrality. The second is to use this "ready" mind to improve your health.

Biofeedback

Biofeedback uses technology to teach you how to develop certain body responses that may help reduce your pain. During a biofeedback session, a trained therapist applies electrodes and other sensors to various parts of your body. The electrodes are attached to devices that monitor and give you feedback on body functions, including muscle tension, brain wave activity, respiration, heart rate, blood pressure and temperature.

Once the electrodes are in place, the therapist uses relaxation techniques to calm you, reducing muscle tension and slowing your heart rate and breathing. You then learn how to produce these changes yourself. The goal of biofeedback is to help you enter a relaxed state in which you can better cope with your pain. Sometimes, specific muscle groups are monitored to help you learn how to position yourself in order to reduce muscle strain.

Biofeedback is, for the most part, widely used and accepted. It has the poten-

tial to improve symptoms associated with many medical conditions. It has relatively few risks, and it's practiced in many medical centers. Studies indicate it has the potential to improve symptoms of headache, anxiety, stress, irritable bowel syndrome and high blood pressure, in addition to improving symptoms of other conditions, such as asthma, nausea and vomiting associated with chemotherapy and incontinence. Research is ongoing.

Hypnosis

People have been using hypnosis to promote healing since ancient times. Hypnosis produces an induced state of relaxation in which your mind stays narrowly focused and open to suggestion. It's not known how hypnosis works, but experts believe it alters your brain wave patterns in much the same way as other relaxation techniques.

For treatment of chronic pain, you receive suggestions designed to help you decrease your perception of the pain and increase your ability to cope with it. Unlike situations sometimes portrayed in movies and on TV, you can't be forced under hypnosis to do something you normally wouldn't want to do.

The success of hypnosis depends on your understanding of the procedure and your willingness to try it. You need to be strongly motivated to change. About 80 percent of adults can be hypnotized by a trained professional. People who don't want to feel out of control often can't be hypnotized.

The National Institutes of Health cites evidence that supports the effectiveness of hypnotherapy in the treatment of chronic pain associated with cancer, irritable bowel syndrome, temporal mandibular joint (TMJ) problems and some types of headache. Studies also show that hypnosis may reduce anxiety. Particularly, hypnosis has been shown to lower anxiety before some medical and dental procedures.

Meditation

The term *meditation* refers to a group of techniques, many of which have their roots in Eastern religious or spiritual traditions. Today, many people use meditation for health and wellness purposes.

In meditation, a person focuses attention on his or her breathing, or on repeating a word, phrase or sound in order to suspend the stream of thoughts that normally occupies the conscious mind. Meditation is believed to lead to a state of physical relaxation, mental calmness, alertness and psychological balance. Practicing meditation can change how you respond to your brain's constant flow of emotions and thoughts, and it may help control how you react to a challenging situation.

Meditation may be practiced on its own or as a part of another mind-body therapy, such as yoga or tai chi. Like these other therapies, once you learn how, you can meditate by yourself.

Meditation may be used to treat a number of problems, including anxiety, pain, depression, stress and insomnia. It can be the perfect complement to the rush of a busy, complicated life. As evidence supporting the use of meditation grows, adding it to your daily schedule may be just the antidote you need to deal with a hectic routine. In addition, if meditation helps lower your blood pressure and reduce stress, so much the better. The long-term benefits of meditation continue to be studied.

Music therapy

Practitioners of music therapy claim that it can lower stress, reduce symptoms of depression and promote pain relief. Like other forms of relaxation, performing or listening to music may help reduce pain by relieving muscle tension and slowing your breathing. Music therapy hasn't been extensively researched, and the few studies published show contradictory findings. However, it poses virtually no risk and is an inexpensive form of therapy. Several organizations promote the use of music for health and healing.

Tai chi

Tai chi (TIE chee), a form of martial arts developed in China, is a popular method for strengthening muscles, improving joint flexibility and reducing stress.

Tai chi involves gentle, deliberate circular movements, combined with deep breathing. As you concentrate on the motions of your body, you develop a feeling of tranquility. For this reason, tai chi is sometimes described as a form of moving meditation. Similar to other forms of Chinese medicine, it's designed to foster the free flow of chi necessary for health.

If you're trying to improve your general health, you may find tai chi helpful

as part of your program. It is generally safe for people of all ages and levels of fitness. Studies show that for older adults it can improve balance and reduce the risk of falls.

Because the movements are low impact and they put minimal stress on your muscles and joints, tai chi is appealing to many. For these same reasons, if you have a condition such as arthritis or you're recovering from an injury, you may find tai chi useful. It may help you reduce your level of stress and manage conditions such as high blood pressure and depression.

Yoga

People practice yoga for many reasons. For some, it's a spiritual path. For others, it's a way to promote physical flexibility, strength and endurance. In either case, you may find that yoga can help you relax and manage stress.

The ultimate goal of yoga is to reach complete peacefulness of body and mind by way of breathing, meditation and posture. Traditional yoga philosophy also requires that practitioners adhere to behavior and dietary practices. However, chances are you may not be looking for a complete change in

lifestyle but rather a tool to help increase flexibility, promote relaxation or relieve stress.

According to the National Institutes of Health, yoga can help reduce stress, slow breathing, lower blood pressure and alter brain waves. Its quiet, precise movements focus your mind less on your busy day and more on the moment at hand, as you move your body through poses that require balance and concentration.

Part 3

Managing chronic pain

Chapter 11

Developing a pain control program

Many people with chronic pain enjoy active and productive lives. If you aren't among them, there's no reason you can't be. But it's up to you to make it happen.

In this chapter and those that follow, we discuss various steps that you can take to help lessen your pain and make it more manageable. There aren't any quick fixes for chronic pain. And most often, you're the key ingredient. If you want your life to improve, you need to lead the way.

You may not like the fact that you have chronic pain. No one does. But clinging to unrealistic hopes or expectations will only prolong your frustra-tion and contribute to your feelings of helplessness.

The first and most important step in controlling chronic pain is accepting the fact that you may always have pain. While some people are able to significantly reduce or eliminate their pain, for many people it will always be a part of their lives. Managing chronic pain is about learning how to keep your pain at a tolerable level so that you can enjoy life.

The remainder of this book focuses on specific lifestyle issues and pain management strategies that can help you better understand and manage your pain. The task ahead may seem daunting, but each small step you take in your new role as pain manager will boost your self-confidence and strengthen your faith in your abilities. The choice is yours to make. You can continue to dwell on your discomfort, or you can do something about it.

Start with SMART goals

Goal setting is an important part of your pain control program, and your first step in achieving pain relief. Goals help divert your attention from your pain, and they provide an opportunity to think about your lifestyle and what you can do to better manage your pain. Goals also give you something to strive for.

But goal setting isn't as easy as it may sound. You simply can't identify some things that you want to occur and expect them to happen. You'll only be setting yourself up for disappointment.

In this chapter we talk about setting SMART goals — goals that are **s**pecific, **m**easurable, **a**ttainable, **r**ealistic and **t**imely. And in the remaining chapters, we give examples of how you can use the SMART formula in various aspects of your pain program.

Specific. Your goals should be clear and straightforward. State exactly what you want to achieve, how you're going to do it and when you want to achieve it. To begin with, set goals that you can achieve within a week to a month. It's easy to give up on goals that take too long to reach. If you have a big goal, break it down into a series of smaller weekly or daily goals. After you achieve one of the smaller goals, move on to the next.

Measurable. A goal doesn't do you any good if there's no way of telling whether you've achieved it. "I want to feel better" isn't a good goal because it's not specific and it's difficult to measure. "I want to be able to work eight hours a day" is a better goal because it's specific and measurable.

Attainable. Ask yourself whether the goal is within reasonable reach. Goals that are too far out of your reach you probably won't commit to doing. For instance, completing a marathon may not be an achievable goal if you've never run before. However, completing a 5K run may be attainable.

How to be SMART

Here are examples of goals that follow the SMART formula:

Goal: Reduce my use of over-the-counter pain medications
When I want to achieve it: 2 weeks
How I'm going to do it: Plan my day to include exercise, pace myself at work and take frequent breaks, use relaxation techniques
How I'm going to measure it: Each day, record in my journal the medication I took and how much

Goal: Exercise 40 minutes each day
When I want to achieve it: 4 weeks
How I'm going to do it: Stretch and do strengthening exercises 15 minutes in the morning, walk 10 minutes during my lunch hour, bicycle 15 minutes in the evening
How I'm going to measure it: Record in my journal when I exercised and for how long

Realistic. Is the goal realistic for you? The purpose of a goal is to shift your focus from your pain to your future. But you can't ignore your limitations. Your goals need to be within your capabilities. If you've suffered a serious back injury, a goal of returning to work as a bricklayer may not be realistic. Instead, your goal might be to find a sales job in a related field. Or you might decide to go back to school for training in a new field.

Timely. Set a time frame for your goal. When do you want to achieve it: Next week? In six months? Putting an end date on your goal gives you a clear target to work toward. If you don't set a completion date, there's less reason to make a commitment.

What are your goals?

Think carefully about some short-term or long-term goals that you want to achieve. If you have some in mind, write them down now.

Consider setting SMART goals for yourself in the following areas if you feel that they're aspects of your life that could use some improvement:

• Becoming more physically active
• Learning to better balance work and leisure activities
• Managing your emotions and behaviors
• Reducing daily stress
• Enjoying time with family and friends
• Taking better care of your overall health
• Reducing your use of medication

Put it in writing

As you begin to think about and set goals, something that you'll find helpful in tracking your progress is a daily journal (see "Sample journal" on page 148). In addition, a journal can help you determine those therapies or activities that seem to be helping you the most. As you work on your goals and you learn techniques to manage your pain, you should see a decrease in your pain level.

A journal can also open your eyes to aspects of your daily life that may be contributing to your pain. Many people think that their pain isn't influenced by factors such as work, stress, sleep or physical activity. But after a few months of tracking their pain levels and their activities, they begin to notice some common patterns.

In addition, a journal can be a great way to express your feelings about your pain or other things that are happening in your life. Writing your thoughts and feelings on paper helps you organize and sort through problems and emotions and get them off your chest, similar to the way you feel after a good heart-to-heart visit with a friend or family member.

Here are things to consider keeping track of in your journal. You don't need to go into a lot of detail if you don't want to. Your journal can be as basic or as detailed as you want it to be.

Pain level and activities

In your journal, begin by recording your pain level. Health care professionals typically measure pain on a scale of 0 to 10, with 0 indicating no pain and 10 being the worst pain imaginable. Using this scale as your guide, rate your pain level and record it in your journal a couple of times a day.

You can do this whenever it's convenient, but keep the times consistent. Many people choose to record their pain level in the morning when they wake up, after lunch and then again in the evening before going to bed.

Keeping a log of your pain levels and activities allows you to:

Learn your pain pattern. Most people find that the changes in their pain levels are quite consistent. For example, your pain may generally be at its lowest level in the morning and its highest level in the evening. Recording your pain levels helps you determine your pain pattern.

Link your pain with your activities. If your pain is the worst in the evening, why? Look to see if certain activities seem to correlate with an increase or a decrease in your pain level. Are you sitting or standing too long? Is your rush to get dinner ready a contributing factor? Are you just tired?

Identify flares. Recording your pain levels helps draw attention to inconsistencies. If your pain level at noon is normally a 3 and one day it's a 6,

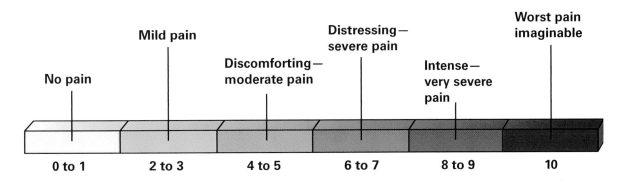

Pain scale

Use this scale as a guide when determining your level of pain.

Sample journal

There is no right or wrong way when it comes to keeping a journal. Some people simply like to jot down their thoughts, and others prefer a worksheet format. This is just one example of how your journal might look and the information to include.

Date: January 1   Hours slept: 7

	7:00 a.m.	1:00 p.m.	10:00 p.m.
Pain level	5	4	6
Mood	7	6	4

Morning

5:00-5:30 Coffee and breakfast
5:30-7:00 Exercised and got ready for work
7:30-11:00 Work
11:30-12:30 15-minute walk and lunch

Afternoon and evening

12:30-4:30 Work
5:00-5:30 Read paper and went through mail
5:30-6:00 Relaxation exercises
6:00-7:00 Dinner
7:00-8:30 Did errands and attended meeting
9:00-10:00 Wrote in journal and got ready for bed.

Comments/thoughts:

I slept a little better last night. I still woke up at 5:00 but I didn't feel so tired. I also seem to have more energy at work. I think the morning exercises are helping. Evenings are still a problem. I know I need to rest more but it seems there are just too many things to do.

seeing the difference may prompt you to think about your morning. Did you do something different?

See your progress. If you feel you aren't making progress, reading your journal may help you to realize that your life has improved, even though the process may seem slow.

Mood

On a scale of 0 to 10, with 0 being poor and 10 being excellent, rate your mood throughout the day. This exercise helps you realize that even though your pain and your mood are closely aligned, they aren't bound together. Typically, the worse your pain, the worse your mood, and vice versa. As you begin to feel more in control of your pain, you may find your mood improving at a faster rate than the improvement in your pain levels. You begin to realize that even though you may not be able to eliminate your pain, you can learn to live with it and still be happy.

Sleep

A good night's sleep better equips you to handle your day. However, getting enough sleep can be difficult because your pain may keep you up at night. In contrast, some people spend too much time in bed. This can also reduce your pain tolerance.

Each day, record how many hours you slept during the night. Eight hours is about average, but the amount of sleep each person needs varies. Your goal should be to feel rested when you wake up. If you're having trouble sleeping, tips to help you sleep better are discussed in Chapter 17.

Going forward

The chapters that follow are devoted to specific components of a pain control program. They include topics such as staying physically active, reducing stress, finding a healthy balance of work and leisure activities, and dealing with difficult emotions and behaviors.

In these chapters, you'll learn about specific steps that you can take to help relieve your pain and improve daily functioning. As you read through these chapters, keep in mind how the two key components outlined here — goal setting and daily journaling — can help you be successful in your efforts to enjoy life with less pain.

Finding the right doctor

Taking charge of your pain doesn't mean that you shouldn't seek help from others. Having people who can help you when you have questions or need assistance is important. A doctor can be especially helpful. But make sure it's a doctor who understands your condition and believes in what you're doing.

The right doctor for you could be your family physician or a specialist who's overseeing your condition. Or you may want to see a doctor or a psychologist who specializes in pain management. If you're not sure where to find a pain specialist, ask your primary care doctor to refer you to one. Before selecting a new doctor, however, check with your health insurance provider to make sure that the care will be covered under your policy.

When selecting a doctor, look for someone who:
- Is knowledgeable about chronic pain
- Wants to help
- Listens well
- Makes you feel at ease
- Encourages you to ask questions
- Seems honest and trustworthy
- Allows you to disagree
- Is willing to talk with your family or friends

In addition to finding the right doctor, make an effort to learn all that you can about your condition and your pain. This will make it easier for the two of you to work together as a team.

Chapter 12

Staying active with daily exercise

There was a time when people with chronic pain were told to avoid physical activity for fear it would damage their joints and muscles and worsen their pain.

A common misconception is that exercise aggravates pain. To the contrary, exercise can help reduce it. During physical activity, your body releases specific chemicals (endorphins and enkephalins) that block pain signals from reaching your brain. These chemicals also help alleviate anxiety and depression, conditions that can make your pain more difficult to control. Exercise also strengthens muscles and ligaments, reducing stress on painful joints.

However, many people bothered by chronic pain don't exercise. Perhaps you tried exercising, but when you did so, the next day your pain was worse so you quit. This is commonly referred to as the "crash and burn" experience. When you first begin to exercise, your pain may worsen for a few days before it improves. The key is to increase your activity level gradually and make exercise a daily habit. With time, you'll have less pain and feel better about yourself.

In the pages that follow, you'll read about specific types of exercise that can help improve your activity level and, in turn, reduce your pain. The exercises fall into three categories:

- Exercises to improve flexibility
- Exercises to improve aerobic capacity
- Exercises to build strength

This fitness plan is safe for almost everyone. However, you still may want to discuss it with your doctor to make sure there aren't any exercises that you should avoid because of a physical condition or injury.

As you begin the program, remember to take it slow and gradually increase your level of activity. Don't try to do too much too soon. Flexibility and aerobic exercises can be done daily, or most days of the week. Include strengthening exercises at least three days a week. If your goal is to build strength in a weakened or painful joint, include strengthening exercises in your routine five days a week.

Before you get started

It's always a good idea to talk with your doctor before starting any type of physical activity program. If you have another health problem or you're at risk of cardiovascular disease, you may need to take some precautions while you exercise.

It's especially important that you see your doctor if you:
- Have a blood pressure of 160/100 millimeters of mercury or higher
- Have diabetes or heart, lung or kidney disease
- Are a man age 40 or older or a women age 50 or older and haven't had a recent physical examination
- Have a family history of heart-related problems before age 55
- Are unsure of your health status
- Have previously experienced chest discomfort, shortness of breath or dizziness during exercise or strenuous activity

Flexibility exercises

Flexibility exercises include range-of-motion and stretching exercises. They ease movement in your joints, allowing you to carry out daily activities more comfortably. They also prevent your muscles from shortening and tightening, which can increase risk of injury.

Range-of-motion exercises

Include some or all of the exercises on the following pages in your physical activity program. With each exercise, move slowly and easily. Repeat each exercise five times, and then move on to the next.

Neck

- Bring your chin toward your chest. Then return to normal position. Avoid extending your neck too far back, as this can worsen neck pain.
- Tilt your left ear toward your left shoulder. Return to normal position and tilt your right ear toward your right shoulder. Avoid raising your shoulder toward your head.

- Turn your face to the left, then to the right. Keep your neck, shoulders and trunk straight.

Jaw

- Open your mouth as wide as possible without clicking or popping. Close.
- Move your jaw to the right, then to the left.
- Move your jaw forward, then back.

Shoulders

With your arms at your sides:
- Roll your shoulders forward in a circular motion. Reverse.
- Bring your arms forward and over your head. Keep your trunk straight.
- Raise your arms from your sides to over your head. Keep your trunk straight and your palms up.
- Bring your elbows to shoulder height. Pull your elbows backward and feel a stretch in your chest muscles.

Elbows

- Bend and straighten your elbows.
- Keeping your arms next to your body, bend your elbows to make a

right angle and turn your palms up
and down.

Wrists

- Move your hands from side to
  side as far as possible, bending
  at the wrists.
- Move your hands up and down,
  bending at the wrists.

Fingers and thumbs

- Bend your fingers to make a fist.
  Then fully straighten them.
- Bend your fingers at the knuckles,
  forming a claw. Then straighten
  them.
- Bend your thumbs across your
  palms and pull toward your
  little fingers.
- Touch the tips of your thumbs to
  the tips of your little fingers. Open
  your hands wide. Repeat, touching
  your thumb to each finger.

Hips

- March in place, bringing your knees
  up high.
- Raise your leg out to the side.
  Alternate legs.
- Lift your leg backward, keeping
  your knee straight. Alternate legs.

- Kick your feet up behind you by
  bending your knees.

Trunk

Standing with your hands on your hips:
- Bend your upper body to the left.
  Repeat to the right.
- Twist your upper body to the right.
  Repeat to the left. Don't turn your
  pelvis.

Ankles and feet

Standing with your feet about 12
inches apart:
- Rise on the toes of both feet. Relax
  to starting position. Rise on the toes
  of your right foot. Relax. Rise on
  the toes of both feet. Relax. Rise on
  the toes of your left foot. Relax.
- Walk on your heels.
- Walk on your toes.
- Walk heel-to-toe, as though you're
  on a tightrope.

Stretching exercises

Stretching each time you exercise helps
to keep your muscles limber and to
reduce tightness in the muscles.

Stretch slowly, holding the position for 30 to 60 seconds, and then slowly release. Breathe deeply and slowly while you stretch. Never bounce, and stretch only until you feel a noticeable pull. Your muscles respond to over-stretching by tightening — the opposite of what you want.

Heel cord stretch (1). Stand at arm's length from a wall with your palms flat against the wall. Keep one leg back with your knee straight and your heel flat on the floor. Slowly bend your elbows and front knee as you lean toward the wall. Hold. Repeat with other leg.

Hamstring stretch (2). Sit on a low table or a chair with your leg propped on another chair in front of you. Without bending your knees, lean forward from your hips. Keep your back straight. Lean forward until you feel a gentle pull in the muscles under your thighs. Hold. Repeat with other leg.

Quadriceps stretch (3). Stand facing a wall or another support. Place your right hand against the wall or on the support. Grasp the top of your left foot with your left hand and gently pull your foot or heel up toward your buttocks until you a feel mild tension in the front of your thigh. Hold your abdomen in and keep your back straight. Hold the stretch and repeat the movement with the other leg. This exercise may also be done while holding on to the back of a chair in front of you with both hands and then pulling a foot up toward your buttock (or as close as you can get) without holding on to the foot. Consider this if balancing on one foot is difficult.

Hip flexor stretch (4). Lie on a low table or a bed with your right leg and hip near the edge. Pull your left thigh and knee firmly toward your chest until your lower back flattens against the table or bed. Let your right leg hang in a relaxed position over the edge of the table or bed. Hold. Repeat with the other leg.

Low back stretch (5). Lie flat on a firm surface. With your knees bent, lift one leg at a time toward your shoulders. Stop when you feel a stretch in your lower back. Return legs one at a time to the starting position. Repeat. Avoid this exercise if you have osteoporosis or have undergone hip replacement.

4

5

Aerobic exercises

Aerobic exercises place added demands on your heart, lungs and muscles, increasing your heart rate, blood pressure and need for oxygen. These exercises help your body work more efficiently and reduce your risk of cardiovascular disease, including heart attack and high blood pressure.

Aerobic activity also increases your stamina, so you don't become as easily fatigued and you have more energy for daily activities.

Aim for 30 to 40 minutes of moderately intense aerobic activity five days each week. You can do this by walking 10 minutes at a time, three times a day. If you've been inactive, start out slowly and gradually increase your time and level of exertion.

There are many types of aerobic activity. Walking is the most common because it's easy to do, convenient and

Looking for a helping hand?

For help with designing and getting started on an activity program, contact one of these professionals:

Physical therapist. A physical therapist is trained in the use of exercise to achieve physical fitness. He or she can help you select the most appropriate exercises based on the location of your pain and show you how to do the exercises properly. While a physical therapist can guide you, it's still up to you to do the exercises.

Occupational therapist. An occupational therapist can teach you how to perform daily activities — such as lifting, reaching and even getting dressed — in ways that won't place extra stress on your joints.

Certified exercise therapist. Many health clubs have employees who are trained in exercise therapy. If you belong to a health club — or are thinking of joining one — make an appointment to meet with a certified therapist for help with developing an exercise plan.

inexpensive. All you need is a good pair of walking shoes.

Other aerobic exercises include:
- Aerobic dance
- Bicycling
- Cross-country skiing
- Dancing
- Golfing
- Hiking
- Snowshoeing
- Swimming and water aerobics

Water aerobics has become increasingly popular among people with chronic pain because water's buoyancy reduces stress on your joints. Water also provides resistance to increase the benefits of aerobic activity. In addition, many people find warm water to be relaxing and soothing to sore muscles and joints.

A disadvantage of water exercises is that they aren't weight bearing. To maintain bone mass and protect against osteoporosis, combine water exercises with activities such as walking or lifting weights.

Strengthening exercises

Strong muscles improve your physical fitness and reduce fatigue. They also make it easier to carry out more vigorous types of daily activities, such as

What about weightlifting?

Lifting weights is an excellent way to strengthen your muscles. However, it's best to work with a physical therapist or fitness trainer in developing and beginning a weightlifting program. A therapist or trainer will help you select the appropriate weights for your level of fitness and teach you how to lift them properly to avoid injury to your muscles and joints.

carrying laundry up and down stairs
or lifting items at work.

To build muscle, include some or
all of these exercises five days a week.
If you're out of shape, begin with five
repetitions of each and slowly build
to 25 repetitions.

Abdominal exercises

**Lie on the floor or on a table, with
your knees bent (6).** Raise your
head and shoulders so that your shoulder blades lift off the floor or table.
Keep your head in a neutral position.
Hold for one or two seconds. Bring
your head and shoulders back down.

**Repeat, reaching both hands toward
your left knee (7).** Relax and repeat
with the right knee. Skip this exercise
if it bothers your neck.

**Lie on a firm surface with your knees
bent (8).** Flatten the small of your back
against the surface and concentrate on
tightening your abdominal muscles.
Relax and repeat.

**Lie on your back with your right
knee bent and your left knee straight
(9).** Hold your abdominal muscles
tight and slowly lower and raise your

6

7

8

left leg. Relax and repeat. Reverse legs. Avoid doing abdominal exercise if you have osteoporosis.

Back exercises

Sit upright in a chair (10). Put your hands on your hips or behind your back and pull your shoulder blades together. Hold for five seconds. Relax and repeat.

Lie facedown over a large pillow with a folded towel under your forehead. Position the pillow under your bellybutton to keep your spine in a neutral position (11). Place your hands at your sides. Pulling your shoulder blades together, raise your head and chest. Keep your neck relaxed. Return to the starting position and repeat. Don't arch.

Leg exercises

Set up two chairs, one in front of the other (12). Hold on to the back of the chair in front of you and begin to sit in the chair behind you. When you get partway down, stop briefly. Return to standing and repeat. This exercise is sometimes referred to as the "minisquat."

Sit back in a chair. Weave a belt around your legs just above your knees so that it forms a figure eight (13). Pulling your legs in opposite directions, lift one leg off the floor. Relax. Repeat with other leg.

Sit far back on a table or in a chair. Weave a belt around your ankles so that it forms a figure eight (14). Try to straighten one leg while pulling the other foot backward, applying equal force with both legs. Gently push for 3 to 5 seconds. Relax. Repeat with the other leg.

Chest and arm exercises

Sit in a sturdy chair that has arms (no wheels), with your feet firmly on the floor. Place your hands on the arms. Push your body up off the surface of the chair using your arms only, not your feet (15). Relax and return to your seat. Repeat.

Stand facing a wall, far enough away that you can place your palms on the wall with your elbows slightly bent (16). Slowly bend your elbows and lean toward the wall. Straighten your arms and return to a standing position. Repeat. As you build strength, try standing farther from the wall.

12

13

14

Perfecting your posture

Good posture places only minimal strain on your joints and muscles. Poor posture, however, can increase stress on some muscles, stretching them or causing them to shorten. When overstretched, your muscles lose their strength and are more prone to injury and pain.

Avoid poor posture
One extreme of poor posture is the swayback (left illustration). In this position, your stomach protrudes too far in front and your buttocks extend too far in the rear. Swayback posture puts excessive pressure on your lower back and can contribute to back problems.

The opposite extreme is the slouch (right illustration), in which your shoulders are rolled forward. If you perpetually slouch, muscles in your chest shorten, reducing your flexibility.

Practice good posture
Good posture will help relax your muscles and may reduce your pain. Throughout the day, including while you exercise, try to maintain good posture.

Good standing posture:
Head erect with chin tucked in, chest held high, shoulders relaxed, hips level, knees straight but not locked, feet parallel.

Good sitting posture:
Spine and head erect, back and legs at a 90-degree angle, natural curves in back maintained.

How to make it work

Regular exercise can help you stay active and allow you to continue to enjoy your favorite leisure activities. The difficulty with exercise is to keep it up — to make it a regular part of your daily routine. You need to find ways to stay active and stay motivated. Here are some tips to get you started:

Set some goals

Start with simple goals and then progress to longer range goals. People who can stay physically active for six months usually end up making regular activity a habit. Remember to make your goals realistic and achievable (see page 144). It's easy to get frustrated and give up on goals that are too ambitious.

Have a game plan

Decide what time of the day you're going to exercise, what exercises you're going to do — flexibility, aerobic and strength — and for how long you are going to do each of the exercises. You don't have to do them all at once. For

15

16

Get SMART

Here are examples of exercise goals that follow the SMART formula:

Goal: Strengthen my knees to help reduce the pain

When I want to achieve it: 3 months

How I'm going to do it: Do strengthening exercises each morning, start
with 15 minutes and build up to 30 minutes

How I'm going to measure it: Each day, record in my journal when I
exercised and for how long and rate the level of pain in my knees

Goal: Have more energy

When I want to achieve it: 4 weeks

How I'm going to do it: Walk for 15 minutes seven days a week and build
up to 30 minutes daily

How I'm going to measure it: Record each day in my journal how long
I exercised

instance, you might do 15 minutes of flexibility exercises in the morning, take a short break and then walk for 20 minutes. In the afternoon, make time for 15 minutes of strengthening exercises.

Don't try to be a jock

The most common mistakes people make are starting an exercise program at too high an intensity and progressing too quickly. The resulting pain and stiffness the next day can be very discouraging. It's better to progress slowly and stay within your capacity.

Shake it up

Vary what you do to prevent boredom. For example, try alternating walking and bicycling with swimming or a low-impact aerobic dance class. On days when the weather is pleasant, do your flexibility or stretching exercises outside.

Put it in writing

To begin with, record what you do each time you exercise, how long you do it, and how you feel during and after exercising. Logging your efforts helps you work toward your goals and reminds you that you're making progress.

Give yourself a pat on the back

After each exercise session, take two to five minutes to relax. Think about what you've just accomplished. This type of internal reward can help you make a long-term commitment to regular exercise.

Chapter 13

Finding balance: Planning and moderation

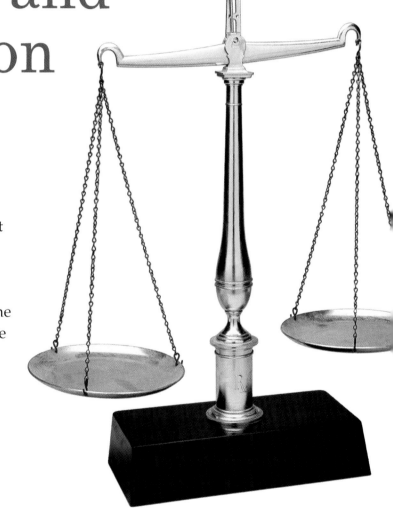

How you organize and go about your day can significantly affect your ability to manage your pain. If you overdo it to meet a deadline at work or overcommit yourself so that you're running from one activity to the next, your body reaches a point where it can't keep up. Fatigue and frustration set in and your pain increases. This can keep you from doing other things that are equally important, such as spending time with family and friends, or having quiet time for yourself.

An unbalanced day

A balanced day

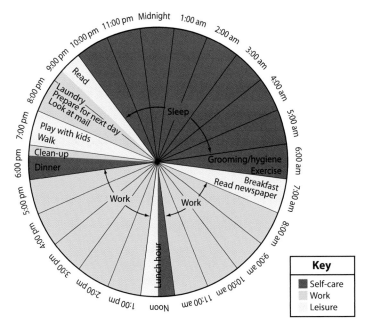

The opposite isn't any better — avoiding daily activities and spending hours lying around the house. The isolation that this lifestyle produces can cause you to focus only on your pain.

The answer is a day that includes a healthy balance — time for work, socializing with family and friends, recreation, hobbies, relaxation and rest. Achieving such a balance can be difficult. You may have a lot of commitments and responsibilities and it isn't easy to change old habits. Instead of drastically altering your daily routine so that it feels uncomfortable, take it one small step at a time. Each week, try to incorporate several small changes. Over time, you'll achieve the balance that's right for you.

How does your day balance out?

Think of how you spend a typical weekday. Does it include a balance of activities? The top circle on the opposite page shows imbalance. Work consumes most of this person's daytime hours, leaving little time for other activities. The bottom example shows a more balanced day that includes time for exercise and relaxation. A healthy balance incorporates time for being productive, as well as resting and having fun.

During the week and on the weekends, try not to spend a disproportionate amount of time on any one activity, such as more than eight hours at work. Instead, aim to include as many activities in your day as feels comfortable. Also make sure to include adequate time for rest.

Put time on your side

For many people, an important step to balancing their day is learning to use time more efficiently. Juggling work, household tasks and social activities can consume large amounts of your day. Procrastination, perfectionism or overcommitting yourself can make time management even more difficult. Taking charge of your time can have a significant impact on how you feel and how much energy you have.

Following are some strategies that can help you use your time more effectively:

Plan. Schedule your day so that you have time for the things you need to do and those you want to do. Write down all of your activities in a daily planner. Then frequently refer to your planner to make sure you stay on track.

It may also be helpful to place a calendar near your telephone to mark down all of your events and appointments so that they don't come as a surprise and to avoid doubling up on commitments. Using a planner doesn't require rigid scheduling. Rather, it simply provides a framework so that you can control how you spend your time.

Recognize patterns. Notice when you waste time and avoid these time wasters. If you can't avoid them, try to make them productive. For example, while waiting for a doctor's appointment or during your daily train commute, listen to a relaxation tape or balance your checkbook.

Prioritize. If you're involved in many activities that are competing for your time, decide which are the most important and let go of the rest. Be aware that another person's priority doesn't have to be your priority. There are times when your needs come before the needs of others. The consequences

of not taking care of yourself likely will be increased pain and fatigue.

Delegate. On days when you have more to do than you can handle, seek help. Asking for assistance, or allowing others to take responsibility for certain things, doesn't indicate a character weakness or flaw. To the contrary, delegating is an example of good time and energy management.

Evaluate. Think about your day. Are your expectations regarding the number of tasks you can complete in a day realistic?

Educate. Discuss your time needs with those who rely on you the most. If family members, friends or co-workers make unreasonable demands on your time, explain to them that to stay active and healthy you need to pace yourself, and that you're making a conscious effort to live a balanced life.

Daily planner

Planning your day can help you achieve a healthier balance to your daily routine. Include a mix of work, rest, exercise, relaxation and social activities. If you have trouble fitting everything in, ask yourself: What do I have to do today? What would best be done today? What do I want to do today?

Day: Thursday

Date: May 10

	I plan to	I did
6:00 a.m.	Exercise, eat breakfast	Exercised, ate breakfast
7:00 a.m.	Clean up and leave for work	Got ready and went to work
8:00 a.m.	Finish letters from yesterday	Letters
9:00 a.m.	Complete letters	Letters, worked on meeting agenda
10:00 a.m.	Start work on new files	Letters
11:00 a.m.	New files	Started new files
Noon	Meet Susan for lunch	Lunch with Susan
1:00 p.m.	Continue work on files	New files
2:00 p.m.	Department meeting	Meeting
3:00 p.m.	Complete files	Meeting follow-up
4:00 p.m.	Make phone calls, other details	Phone calls, memos, etc.
5:00 p.m.	Go home, rest, ride bike	Went home, rested, rode bike
6:00 p.m.	Prepare and eat dinner	Ate dinner
7:00 p.m.	Do laundry and iron	Laundry, rested
8:00 p.m.	Work on class reunion schedule	Ironed, visited with Louise
9:00 p.m.	Relaxation exercises, rest	Relaxation exercises, helped Jeff
10:00 p.m.	Read book, go to bed	Read book and went to bed
11:00 p.m.	Sleep	Slept

Daily planner

Make photocopies of this page and use the planner to schedule your day. You can plan a day at a time or make your plans for several days. Each day, write down what you did and compare it with your plan. If you find that scheduling your day helps you achieve your goals, then continue to do so.

Day: _____

Date: _____

	I plan to	I did
6:00 a.m.		
7:00 a.m.		
8:00 a.m.		
9:00 a.m.		
10:00 a.m.		
11:00 a.m.		
Noon		
1:00 p.m.		
2:00 p.m.		
3:00 p.m.		
4:00 p.m.		
5:00 p.m.		
6:00 p.m.		
7:00 p.m.		
8:00 p.m.		
9:00 p.m.		
10:00 p.m.		
11:00 p.m.		

Get more organized

Becoming more organized can save you time so that you can incorporate more activities into your day. Organization also helps conserve energy.

Think before you act. Before you begin a task, gather all the items you'll need or make a list. For example, keep all of your cleaning supplies in one bucket to avoid multiple trips up and down the stairs. Make a list before you run errands, to avoid additional trips.

Keep commonly used items accessible. Organize your work areas at home and at your job so that items you use frequently are close at hand. This can save you unnecessary bending or reaching. At home, this might include keeping your spoons and spatulas next to the stove or your wrenches and screwdrivers by your workbench.

Reduce clutter. Searching for items takes time and energy. Organize your counters, drawers and closets so that you can easily find what you need. Don't let housework and paperwork pile up.

Do everything in moderation

Moderation involves how much, how long or how fast you do things to avoid overdoing or underdoing activities during your day. By moderating activities, you can improve your ability to accomplish daily tasks without increasing pain levels or fatigue. To practice moderation:

Break apart lengthy tasks. Lengthy activities often deplete your energy and may increase your pain. Instead of spending all day Saturday planting your garden, spend an hour or two in the garden over three or four days. Another example is to divide a 10-hour car trip to visit relatives into two days instead of one. Get out and stretch every 90 minutes or 90 miles.

Alternate activities. Mix activities that require a lot of effort with those that require only a little energy. After vacuuming one room of the house, sit down and fold laundry. After mowing the lawn, read or watch a movie.

Prioritize tasks. Note those times of the day when you have the most energy. Plan your priority tasks — those chores you "have to" get done — during these times.

Take frequent rest breaks. How often you should take a break depends on the activity. You may find that you can do some activities, such as word processing, for 30 minutes to an hour before you need a break. More strenuous tasks, such as mowing the lawn or cleaning the house, may require a break every 10 to 20 minutes. It's important to take a break before you become fatigued.

Work at a moderate pace. Instead of rushing to complete a task, take your time and work at a comfortable speed — one at which you feel like you're exerting yourself but not overdoing it. You expend twice as much energy when you work at a fast pace compared with a moderate one. It may take you a little longer to get the job done, but in the end you'll feel better.

Change the frequency of tasks. Some tasks may be less fatiguing if you break them up and do them more often. For example, try doing your laundry three times a week with smaller loads rather than spending several hours on one day doing the chore.

Develop better daily habits

Do you always stand at the kitchen counter while chopping vegetables? Do you balance on your tiptoes to reach items on high shelves? Do you sit while reading through correspondence at work? If so, do you know why? Chances are, it's because that's the way you've always done it.

Adding balance to your day also involves looking for new and more efficient ways to perform everyday tasks. You want to avoid reaching, bending, twisting or prolonged sitting or standing, actions that consume energy and that can aggravate your pain. For example, instead of standing to chop up vegetables, pull up a stool or sit at the kitchen table. Instead of stretching to reach an item on a high shelf, use a footstool. Instead of always sitting at your desk while you read, walk around your office.

The less tired you are from doing simple things, the more energy you'll have for more strenuous tasks. Here are examples of some simple ways you can modify your day.

While getting dressed

- Gather all articles of clothing.
- Sit down to put on your clothes.
- Place your foot on a chair or stool when tying your shoes.
- Avoid clothes that button or tie in the back.

In the kitchen

- Bend your knees, not your back, to reach items on lower shelves.
- Place one foot on a footstool when standing for long periods, and alternate feet.
- Organize cupboards to keep frequently used items within reach.

- Store heavy items at waist level.
- Use electrical appliances when possible, such as an electric can opener.
- Choose quick and easy recipes or double recipes and freeze extra portions for another day's meal.

Around the house

- Use a long-handled duster for hard-to-reach corners and a long-handled mop to clean your floors.
- Use your legs, not your arm, to move the vacuum cleaner.
- Sit on a stool to remove laundry from your dryer.
- Position your bed so that you have access to it from three sides. When

making your bed, get on your knees to tuck in bed sheets and blankets. Instead of lifting the mattress, push the sheets and blankets between the mattress and box spring.

When outdoors

- Use a wheeled cart to move heavy items.
- Mow your lawn with a self-propelled mower.

- Purchase power tools, such as a nail driver and screwdriver.
- Use tools or assistive devices that reduce strain on your joints, such as garden or yard tools with enlarged grips.
- Use a long-handled rake or hoe to avoid bending.
- Bend your knees when shoveling snow, and use your legs to slide the snow and lift the load. Use a small, lightweight shovel.

Don't hold your breath

If you've been in an exercise class, you may have heard your instructor say, "Don't forget to breathe." And you may have said to yourself, "Of course I'm breathing."

It's common to hold your breath when you're concentrating on an activity, such as exercising, or struggling with a simple task, such as opening a lid on a jar. And often, you don't even realize that you're doing it. When you hold your breath, however, you limit oxygen to your muscles just when they need it the most. Because your muscles can't perform to their capacity without adequate oxygen, you become more easily fatigued.

To keep from holding your breath, exhale when you exert the most energy, such as twisting a jar lid or lifting a heavy box from the floor. Your body will naturally respond by breathing in.

Move your body wisely

Changing how you perform daily activities is based on using your muscles and joints correctly. Proper body mechanics begin with good posture. When you stand or sit, try to keep your shoulders and neck relaxed and your spine aligned properly.

If you sit for prolonged periods, occasionally elevate your legs by placing your feet on a footstool. Also change positions to shift your weight. This helps divert stress to different muscles. The same strategies apply to prolonged standing. Shift your weight to change positions and use a footstool.

Here are some examples of other proper ways to move your body when performing basic tasks.

Reaching

- Avoid excessive arching and twisting of your back.
- Maintain normal spine curves.
- Place one foot forward as close to the object as possible. Grasp the object and pull it slowly to the edge

of the shelf by shifting your body weight to your back foot.

- Slowly lower the object to waist level, using your arms. Keep the object as close to you as possible.

Pushing

- Bend your knees so that your arms are level with the object.
- Maintain normal spine curves and walk, using your legs to push the object ahead of you.

Pulling

- Bend your knees so that your arms are level with the object.
- Maintain normal spine curves and walk backward, pulling the object with your whole body weight instead of just your arms or back.
- If possible, push the object rather than pull it.

Kneeling

- Keep your feet 8 to 12 inches apart.
- Place one foot forward and lower your body to one knee, keeping your weight on the balls of your feet.
- If you need, use your arms to help you move in and out of a kneeling position.

- Maintain normal spine curves.
- To progress to full kneeling, lower yourself until both knees are on the floor, and sit back on your heels.
- Reverse the process to stand.

Lifting

- Follow the steps for kneeling, making sure you stand close to the object you're going to lift.
- If the object is heavy, lift it first to your bent knee.
- Lift using your leg muscles to rise from the floor.
- Carry the object close to your body at about waist level. If possible, place your forearms under the object.
- Turn by pivoting your feet. Don't twist at your waist.

Using long-handled tools

- Stand with one foot forward and use a rocking motion. During the forward stroke, shift your body weight to your forward foot. When you pull back, shift your weight to your back foot.
- Use arm and leg movements instead of back movements.
- Avoid overreaching and twisting. Use long, smooth strokes.

- Occasionally switch hand positions, exchanging your top hand with your bottom hand.

Get SMART

Here are examples of daily living goals that follow the SMART formula:

Goal: Spend fewer hours at work or doing work activities at home

When I want to achieve it: 4 weeks

How I'm going to do it: Try to leave the office at 5:30 each day, don't stay to "finish up" a task, try not to bring work home

How I'm going to measure it: Record each day in my journal how many hours I spent at work or on work-related tasks at home

Goal: Better organize my day

When I want to achieve it: Next week

How I'm going to do it: Sit down each morning at breakfast and log in my planner what I am going to do that day and stick with the plan, delegate some tasks so that I don't have to spend so much time running errands and rushing around

How I'm going to measure it: Each day, record in my planner what I did and compare it with my plan

Chapter 14

Dealing with your emotions and behaviors

When chronic pain intrudes on your life, you may find yourself overwhelmed by intense, often negative, emotions, including panic, fear, grief and anger. Like the pain that causes them, these emotions can linger and transform you into a different person — a person you don't like.

Changes in your behavior, expressed through words and actions, can affect your sense of self-worth and your relationships. These changes can also affect your body, sapping your energy and intensifying your pain.

But there are positive ways for dealing with these changes. The techniques outlined in this chapter are designed to help you recognize and deal with negative changes, improve relationships and become more effective at managing your pain.

Admitting your loss

For many people, the first step in dealing with negative feelings is to admit that the feelings exist. That's very difficult for some people to do, especially in a culture that often praises the optimist and criticizes the complainer.

If you're grappling with chronic pain, one of the earliest and most wrenching emotions you experience is a deep sense of loss. You may miss:

- The healthy person you once were
- Untroubled family relationships
- Your independence
- Gatherings with friends
- Feelings of energy and confidence
- Job satisfaction
- An enjoyable hobby
- A sense of happiness
- Sexual intimacy

These are difficult losses. You may feel as if you've lost nearly everything precious to you. Your natural response is to grieve.

Feelings associated with grieving

Grieving can trigger a number of different feelings. Many people respond to chronic pain with the same feelings that often accompany the loss of a loved one.

Denial. You may deny you're in pain. You continually seek a cure even though you've been told that your pain is incurable.

Anger or frustration. You've tried numerous ways to control your pain, and nothing seems to be working. You find yourself more irritable more often. You get upset because others don't seem to understand what you're going through.

Depression. Over time, you become overwhelmed by feelings of sadness, worthlessness and helplessness. You don't feel like doing anything — even things you once enjoyed — and you have difficulty concentrating. You withdraw from others.

Guilt and shame. You sense you're not the person you used to be. You feel you're letting down those who are closest to you.

Acceptance. You stop focusing on things you can't change and begin to look to the future. You accept that your pain is a part of your life.

As you work your way through these emotions, consider these suggestions:

- Recognize your losses as serious. Don't trivialize them.
- Admit your feelings to yourself and others — especially supportive family, friends and your doctor. Acknowledging and talking about your feelings is the first step toward emotional health.
- Give yourself time for emotional healing, and ask your doctor, a counselor or a therapist for advice and help.

Dealing with depression

Depression is a medical disorder that affects your thoughts, moods, feelings, behavior and even your physical health. Depression and chronic pain are closely linked. Research suggests that pain and depression share common pathways in the emotional (limbic) region of the brain — which may, in part, explain their association.

Depression can increase your response to pain, or at least increase the severity of your pain. Conversely, chronic pain is stressful and depressing in itself. Sometimes the two create a vicious cycle — your pain makes your depression worse, and the worse your depression the worse your pain.

Two hallmarks of depression — symptoms key to establishing a diagnosis — are:

- Loss of interest in normal daily activities. You lose interest in or pleasure from activities that you used to enjoy.
- Depressed mood. You feel sad, helpless or hopeless, and may have crying spells.

If you think you may be experiencing depression, it's important that you talk to your doctor. Many people with chronic pain don't mention possible depression to their doctors because they figure that as soon as they get treatment for their pain, their

Learning positive self-talk

There are many ways to cope with the upsetting changes and emotions chronic pain can produce. One coping technique is positive self-talk.

Self-talk is the stream of thoughts that run through your head every day. Some people refer to this as automatic thinking. Your automatic thoughts may be positive or negative. Some are based on logic and reason. Others may be misconceptions that you formulate from lack of adequate information.

The goal of positive self-talk is to weed out the misconceptions and challenge them with rational and positive thoughts. The process is simple, but it takes time and practice. Throughout the day, stop and evaluate what you're thinking and find a way to put a positive spin on your negative thoughts. Don't say to yourself anything that you wouldn't say to someone else. If a negative thought enters your mind, evaluate it rationally and respond with affirmations of what's good about yourself. Here are some examples:

Negative or irrational beliefs	Positive or rational beliefs
Because of my pain, I'm no longer the person I was. I'm no longer loved and appreciated.	I'm worthy of love, and I'm worthy of being appreciated for all that I am.
If I go out with friends and my pain acts up, I won't be able to manage. I'll embarrass myself and ruin things for everyone.	I can enjoy friends and have a good time. I may take breaks from my usual activities, but it can still be fun.

Negative or irrational beliefs	Positive or rational beliefs
I have no control over my happiness. Pain controls me.	I can control my happiness. I can enjoy life regardless of pain.
I used to be able to do so many things. Now I can't do anything.	I can do a lot more than I thought. Almost everything I used to do I can still do to some degree.
People at work are upset with me. They think I'm not doing my share of the work.	I will do the best job I can. My co-workers will have to learn to accept my limitations.
Medical science can do so much. Certainly there must be a cure for my pain.	Medical science can't fix every-thing. Many problems aren't cured but controlled.

Types of irrational thinking

Following are some common forms of distorted, negative thinking. A growing amount of research suggests a connection between irrational thinking and increased levels of pain.

Catastrophizing. You automatically anticipate the worst.

Generalizing. You see a specific, troubling event as the beginning of an unending cycle.

Emotionalizing. You let your feelings control your judgment.

Personalizing. When something bad occurs, you automatically think that you're to blame.

Filtering. You magnify the negative aspects of a situation and filter out all of the positive ones.

Polarizing. You see things only as black and white, good or bad. There's no middle ground.

Overcoming irrational thoughts

Life isn't worth living. *Yes, it is. I'll make it through this.*

There's something terribly wrong. *I shouldn't anticipate the worst.*

Because of my pain, I'm stupid and boring. *No, I'm not stupid and boring.*

This isn't fair. Someone should be able to cure my pain. *It may not be fair, but I can deal with it.*

Pain in control
You in control

I can't handle the pain. *Maybe a walk will distract me.*

I can't finish anything anymore. *I don't have to finish everything.*

No one wants to be around me. *I can enjoy time with family and friends. I'll talk less about my pain.*

I should be doing more. I've become a burden. *I'm staying active and doing what I can.*

Pain is my whole life. *Pain is not my entire life. There's more to me than my pain.*

depression will go away. However, to effectively treat your pain, your doctor needs to know that you may also be experiencing depression.

If you're dealing with both chronic pain and depression, it's important that both conditions be treated. A better mood often means reduced pain, and vice versa.

Treatment of depression typically involves medication (see page 90). Some medications used to treat depression, such as tricyclic antidepressants, have also been shown to reduce pain — one drug can help treat both conditions. Just the opposite, some medications used to treat pain may worsen depression. That's why it's important that your doctor know if you may be experiencing depression. Another common treatment for depression is psychotherapy. There are several types of psychotherapy. Each is aimed at helping you identify and deal with one or

more issues that may be contributing to your depression.

Managing your anxiety

It's normal to feel anxious or worried at times. Everyone does. But if you feel anxious all of the time or your anxiety is interfering with your daily life, you need to talk to a doctor.

Like depression, chronic pain and anxiety tend to go hand in hand. When you have chronic pain, you may fear the worst. You may worry about re-injury, your job status and changes in your finances, or increased pain. Such fears contribute to self-limiting behavior and a self-defeating attitude.

A common fear is that your pain will only get worse. This can become a self-fulfilling prophecy. A cycle can develop in which higher anxiety leads to increased pain sensitivity, which leads to more fear and anxiety, which, in turn, results in more pain.

Fortunately, there are ways to treat and break this destructive pattern. The two main treatments for anxiety are medication and psychotherapy. Medications include anti-anxiety drugs, such as sedatives, and anti-depressants (see page 90). Psycho-therapy involves receiving help from a mental health professional through a combination of talking and listening.

A tool that you can use to objectively examine the cause of your fear and anxiety is positive self-talk (see "Learning positive self-talk," page 184). In addition, talk with your doctor or another health professional about your fears and concerns, especially if your anxiety level interferes with your daily functioning.

Managing your anger

Unrelenting pain, interrupted sleep, unsuccessful treatments, job difficulties and insurance battles — there are a lot of things that can make you angry when you're experiencing pain. But it's unhealthy to stay angry, bottle up your anger or express it with explosive outbursts.

And anger isn't always easy to identify. Mild anger can express itself in the form of increased irritability, or being short-tempered or difficult to be around.

Whether it's short term and intense or lingering and subdued, mismanaged anger can hurt you in many ways. Anger can lead to headaches, back-aches, high blood pressure, irritable bowel syndrome and other health problems. Anger can also influence your pain. It typically produces muscle tension, making it difficult to relax.

Here are some ideas to help you man-age your anger:

Identify your anger triggers. For example, if you know that a particular friend often manages to upset you, prepare for the next visit. Think about topics that spark your anger, and practice what to say to defuse the situation. For example, if your friend brings up a past dispute, respond by saying, "Oh, we've discussed that before. Certainly we've got more interesting things to talk about."

Identify symptoms of emerging anger. What do you do when you start to get angry? Do you clench your teeth? Do your neck and shoulders begin to tense up? Read these symptoms like a caution light — a warning that you're getting angry.

Respond to your symptoms. When you find yourself becoming angry, take a short timeout. Count to 10, take a few deep breaths, look out a window — anything to buy yourself some time to let your brain catch up with your emotions and allow you a moment to think before you act.

Give yourself time to cool down. Before you confront the individual who has made you angry, look for a way to release some of your emotional energy. You might go for a walk, visit the gym, clean the house or mow the lawn.

Don't bottle up your anger. Try to deal with disappointment early, before you become extremely angry.

If your anger stems from what someone did or said, talk directly to that person. Deal only with the current situation, and approach it from the perspective of how you feel instead of what the person did. For example, try a statement like this: "I feel hurt by what you said." That way, you're more likely to find a receptive listener than if you launch a blame-offensive statement, such as, "You insulted me for the 20th time today!"

Find release valves. Look for creative ways to release the energy produced by your anger. These might include listening to music, painting or writing in your journal.

Get a new perspective. Anger and frustration can increase when you have unrealistic expectations of others or yourself. If changing your environment isn't possible and assertive communication doesn't help, then changing your expectations may help you gain peace of mind. The bottom line: You can't keep yourself from getting angry, but you can manage your anger so that it doesn't become an ongoing problem.

Changing your expectations

Some people are perfectionists, constantly striving for excellence. These are the homemakers whose house could pass a military white-glove inspection, the master welders who pride themselves on their precision work and the grandparents who never miss their grandchild's soccer games.

This compulsive perfectionism isn't the lifestyle for someone with chronic pain. It's not easy to try and live up to a perfectionist's expectations, and trying to do so can become emotionally and physically damaging.

Before pain invaded your life, perhaps you could work 50 to 60 hours a week with no problem, clean your entire house in two hours and play a set of tennis every Saturday. Now, even part-time work leaves you exhausted, household chores become intimidating, and day long projects and tennis are unimaginable.

As long as you compare yourself with how you used to be, you'll feel miserable about your performance.

Your work won't be good enough, and your leisure time won't be enjoyable enough.

There is, however, a way to keep an upbeat outlook, and that's to become a perfectionist at adjusting your goals. People who don't adapt to new challenges are more likely to become discouraged and depressed. But those who are flexible enough to adjust their expectations generally have a positive attitude about life and manage to stay active. "I can't work a full-time job and still keep a perfect house," you might say to yourself, "but I can at least clean up the dirty dishes in the kitchen and make sure the floors aren't littered with newspapers and clothes."

Instead of focusing on performance and appearance, as perfectionists often do, work on "perfecting" your character to an individual who values inner peace, patience and kindness.

Learning to assert yourself

Responding to all of the challenges of daily life can be difficult. And sometimes, one of the toughest tasks is learning to say no, even when doing so is in your best interest. To keep from disappointing others, you do things you know you shouldn't. You spend all day on your feet shopping with a friend. You agree to stay late at work to finish a last-minute project.

This is passive behavior. You put your thoughts, feelings and health aside for the sake of others. Passive behavior can stem from your upbringing and your beliefs about the importance of helping others and treating them with respect. Or it can result from low self-esteem.

Unfortunately, passive behavior and chronic pain can be a dangerous combination. When you continually give in to the wishes of others — at your expense — your frustration can grow, your self-esteem erode and your pain increase.

Aggressive behavior isn't any better. Contrary to passive behavior, aggressive behavior is being insensitive to others or accomplishing your goals at their expense. Examples include barging ahead of people who are waiting patiently, or voicing your opinions in such a way that you intimidate others from speaking up. Often, aggressive

behavior begins with "you should" statements, which prompt a negative reply that leads to conflict.

So, how do you stand up for yourself without being blunt or hurtful to others? The answer is assertive behavior.

Assertive behavior is honestly and openly expressing your feelings while showing concern for the feelings of others. Here's an example. "I miss spending time with all of you, and I'd like to go golfing with the group. But instead of playing 18 holes, I'm going to stop after nine and wait for you to finish. I hope you can understand."

Assertive behavior is based on I statements. (The word *I* is used four times in the previous paragraph.) I statements tell people how you feel without placing blame or creating feelings of guilt.

Steps to being more assertive

These suggestions can help you be more assertive when communicating with others:

Observe your behavior. Honestly evaluate your behavior when speaking with others. Are there times when you're assertive, or are you always passive or aggressive? Make a mental note of situations in which you felt you responded well and those in which you feel you could have done better.

Think before you respond. When you want to make a statement or you're asked a question, think briefly about the best way to get your point across assertively, instead of simply blurting out an automatic response.

Get SMART

Here are examples of some emotional and behavioral goals that follow the SMART formula:

Goal: Not get so down on myself
When I want to achieve it: 1 month
How I'm going to do it: Try not blame myself for everything that goes wrong, practice positive self-talk, spend more time with positive people and make it a point to see a funny movie when possible
How I'm going to measure it: Record each day in my journal my mood level on a scale of 1-10

Goal: Try not to be such a perfectionist
When I want to achieve it: 3 months
How I'm going to do it: Each day make a list of what has to be done and what can wait until another day, learn to relax when things don't go as planned using relaxation techniques, have someone come in once a month to do a full housecleaning
How I'm going to measure it: Plan my day to include time for relaxation and each day record in my journal my anxiety level

Plan for a difficult situation. Think about a situation you're likely to encounter in which you'll need to be assertive. Close your eyes and imagine how you'll respond. What might the person say? What will you say in return?

Pay attention to your body language. As you practice being more assertive, observe how you stand or sit, along with your gestures, facial expressions and eye contact. For example, when talking to someone, do you look at the person? Or do you stare at the ceiling or floor or out a window?

Boosting your self-esteem

Your struggle with chronic pain can result in some damaging blows to your self-image. Some of these are self-imposed, such as your inability to measure up to your own expectations. Others may come from family, friends, colleagues or even strangers.

It's important to maintain a sense of self-worth. The better you feel about yourself, the better you'll take care of yourself. In addition, a positive self-image has been linked to better health and a stronger immune system. Feeling good about yourself may actually improve your health.

Many of the steps discussed in this chapter — managing your anger, practicing positive thinking, challenging your expectations and learning how to assert yourself — will have a positive effect on your self-esteem. As you learn how to control and express your emotions, you'll feel better about yourself and more confident in your abilities, and your self-image will improve.

There may be days, however, when your self-esteem could use a little energizing. When that happens, consider these suggestions:

Structure your day with goals you can meet. When the day is done, you'll feel a sense of accomplishment.

Spend time with others. Being around people will make you feel more connected and less alone.

Talk with a friend. Having someone who's willing to take time to listen lets you know that you're valued.

Find new friends. Misery loves company, and you may find that some relationships may be negative or even based solely on physical complaints. Make friends with people who have something in common with you as a person, not with people who only share your pain symptoms.

Treat yourself to something you enjoy. Just as you buy gifts for others who are feeling down, you need to do the same for yourself.

Spruce up your appearance. Try a different hairstyle. Buy some new clothes. The better you look, the better you feel about yourself.

List reasons people like you. It reminds you that you have special qualities people enjoy.

List things you do well. Then do one of them.

A healthy sense of self-esteem can improve many aspects of your life.

When you value yourself, you're open to learning and feedback from others, which increases your ability to meet and solve challenges. Because you feel secure and worthwhile, your relationships become more positive.

Responding to your behaviors

In chapter 4, we showed what happens when pain takes control of your behaviors. The illustration on page 195 shows how you can regain control of your behaviors by counteracting the pain with a variety of healthy responses.

Responding to your emotions

In chapter 4, we also showed what happens when pain takes control of your emotions. The illustration on page 196 indicates steps that you can take to regain control of your emotions so that you can enjoy life and not fall into despair and depression.

Behavioral cycle

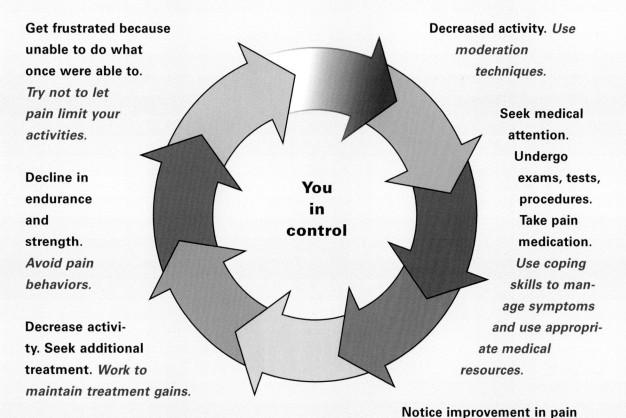

Withdraw and isolate. *Resume family and work roles. Set future goals.*

Get frustrated because unable to do what once were able to. *Try not to let pain limit your activities.*

Decline in endurance and strength. *Avoid pain behaviors.*

Decrease activity. Seek additional treatment. *Work to maintain treatment gains.*

Experience an increase in pain. *Use coping strategies — exercise, relaxation, positive self-talk — to manage pain.*

Experience injury or illness. (Start of pain) *Assess your symptoms.*

Decreased activity. *Use moderation techniques.*

Seek medical attention. Undergo exams, tests, procedures. Take pain medication. *Use coping skills to manage symptoms and use appropriate medical resources.*

Notice improvement in pain level. *Continue to use moderation techniques.*

Increased activity. Overdo it. *Use time management skills and set realistic goals.*

You in control

Emotional cycle

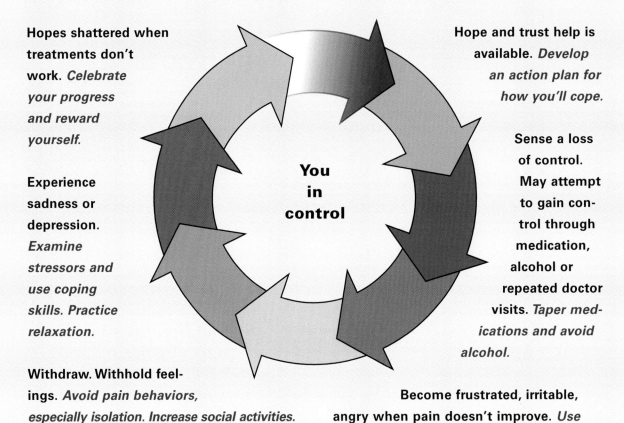

Decrease in self-esteem. *Self-esteem will improve with a sense of accomplishment. Plan for the future.*

Experience fear and anxiety. Focus on the pain. (Start of pain) *Examine recent activities and events.*

Hopes shattered when treatments don't work. *Celebrate your progress and reward yourself.*

Hope and trust help is available. *Develop an action plan for how you'll cope.*

Experience sadness or depression. *Examine stressors and use coping skills. Practice relaxation.*

Sense a loss of control. May attempt to gain control through medication, alcohol or repeated doctor visits. *Taper medications and avoid alcohol.*

You in control

Withdraw. Withhold feelings. *Avoid pain behaviors, especially isolation. Increase social activities.*

Become frustrated, irritable, angry when pain doesn't improve. *Use anger management strategies.*

Feel guilty for behavior. *Work on self-talk and communications skills. Reward yourself for your efforts and progress.*

Chapter 15

Managing stress

Pain and stress go hand in hand. When you're in pain, you're less able to handle the stress of everyday life. Common hassles turn into major obstacles. Stress may also cause you to do things that intensify your pain, such as tense your muscles, grit your teeth and stiffen your shoulders. In short, pain causes stress, and stress intensifies pain.

The first step in breaking this pain-stress cycle is to realize that stress is your response to an event, not the event itself. It's something you can control. That's why events that are stressful for some people aren't for others. For example, your morning commute may leave you anxious and tense because you use it as worry time.

Your co-worker, however, finds her commute relaxing. She enjoys her time alone without distractions. Understanding that you have control over your stress can help you develop positive strategies for dealing with stress.

What stress does to you

When you encounter stress, your body responds in a manner similar to a physical threat. It automatically gears up to face the challenge or musters the strength necessary to get out of trouble's way.

This fight-or-flight response results from the release of hormones that cause your body to shift into overdrive. Your heart beats faster, your blood pressure increases, and your breathing quickens and becomes more shallow. Your nervous system also springs into action, causing your facial muscles to tighten and your body to perspire more.

Stress can be negative or positive:
- Positive stress provides a feeling of excitement and opportunity. Positive stress often helps athletes perform better in competition than in practice. Other examples of positive stress include a new job or the birth of a child.
- Negative stress occurs when you feel out of control or under constant or intense pressure. You may have trouble concentrating, or you may feel alone. Family, finances, work, isolation and health problems, including pain, are common causes of negative stress.

Persistent stress can have a negative effect on your health. In addition to the strain it puts on your cardiovascular system, the hormone cortisol released during stress may suppress your immune system, making you more susceptible to infections and disease. Stress can also cause headaches and worsen intestinal problems and asthma.

What are your stress triggers?

Stress is often associated with situations or events that you find difficult to handle. How you view things also affects your level of stress. If you have unrealistic or high expectations, chances are you'll experience more than your fair share of stress.

Take some time to think about what causes you stress. Your stress may be linked to external factors, such as:

- Work
- Family
- Relationships
- Unpredictable events
- Daily environment
- Community

Stress can also come from internal factors, such as:

- Irresponsible behavior
- Poor health habits
- Negative attitudes and feelings
- Unrealistic expectations
- Perfectionism

Jot down what seem to be sources of stress for you. And then ask yourself if there's anything you can do to lessen the stress or avoid these stressors. Some stressors you can control and some you can't.

Concentrate on stressful events or situations in your life that you can change. For events or situations that are beyond your control, look for ways to adapt — to remain calm under trying circumstances.

How to stress less

It's one thing to be aware of stress in your daily life, but it's another to know how to change it. As you look through your list of stressors, think carefully about why they're so bothersome. For example, if your busy day is a source of stress, ask yourself if it's because you tend to squeeze too many things into your day or because you aren't organized.

The following techniques can help you reduce sources of stress that you can control and better cope with those that you can't.

Change your lifestyle

Consider these changes to your daily routine as ways to help alleviate stress:

Plan your day. This can help you feel more in control of your life. You might start by getting up 15 minutes earlier to ease the morning rush. Do unpleasant tasks early in the day and be done with them. Keep a written schedule of your daily activities so that you're not faced with conflicts or last-minute rushes (see page 171). Because a pain flare-up can happen at any time, have a backup plan — decide what has to be done now and what can wait until later.

Simplify your schedule. Prioritize, plan and pace yourself. Learn to delegate responsibility to others at home and at work. Say no to added responsibilities or commitments if you're not up to doing them. Try not to feel guilty if you aren't productive every moment.

Get organized. Organize your home and work space so that you know where things are. Keep your house, car and personal belongings in working order to prevent untimely and stressful repairs.

Exercise regularly. Regular physical activity helps loosen your muscles and relieves emotional intensity. Try to exercise for at least 30 minutes most days of the week.

Get enough sleep. This can give you the energy you need to face each day. Going to sleep and awakening at a consistent time also may help you sleep more soundly.

Eat well. A diet that includes a variety of healthy foods provides the right mix

Taking a breather

Here's an exercise to help you practice deep, relaxed diaphragmatic breathing. Practice it throughout the day until it becomes natural so that you can use it readily when you feel stressed.

- Lie down on your back or sit comfortably with your feet flat on the floor.
- With your mouth closed and shoulders relaxed, inhale slowly and deeply through your nose to the count of six. Allow the air to fill your diaphragm — the muscle between your abdomen and your chest.
- Pause for a second.
- Slowly exhale the air through your mouth as you count to six.
- Pause for a second.
- Repeat the breathing cycle several times.

You're breathing correctly when your abdomen — not your chest — moves with each breath. If you're lying down, place a paperback book on your abdomen. When you breathe in, the book should rise. When you breathe out, the book should go down.

of nutrients to keep your body systems working well. When you're healthy, you're better able to control stress and pain.

Change the pace. Occasionally break away from your routine and explore new territory without a schedule. Take a vacation, even if it's just a weekend getaway.

Be positive. There's no room for "Yes, but .... ." Avoiding negative self-talk can be difficult. It helps to spend time with people who have a positive outlook and a sense of humor. Laughter actually helps ease pain. It releases endorphins, chemicals in your brain that give you a sense of well-being. If you're feeling stressed, turn on the television or go to the movie theater and enjoy a funny movie.

Stay connected. Recognize when you need the support of family and friends. Talking about your problems with others can often relieve pent-up emotions and lead to solutions you hadn't thought of on your own.

Take breaks. Periodically take time to relax, stretch or walk. Relaxation is a great way to combat the effects of stress.

Learn how to relax

You can't avert all sources of stress, such as an unexpected visit from family or a problem at work. However, you can modify how you react to these situations by practicing relaxation techniques. Relaxation helps relieve stress that can aggravate chronic pain. It also reduces muscle tension. Relaxation won't cure your pain, but it can:

- Reduce anxiety and conserve energy
- Increase your self-control when dealing with stress
- Help you recognize the difference between tense muscles and relaxed ones
- Help you physically and emotionally handle your daily demands
- Help you remain alert, energetic and productive

Keep in mind, though, that the benefits of relaxation are only as good as your efforts. Learning to relax takes time.

Techniques to try

There are many ways to relax. A number of relaxation techniques, such as yoga, meditation, massage and tai chi are discussed in Chapter 10. Following are some other simple tools you can use when you feel stressed. Work on these relaxation techniques at least once or twice a day until they come naturally. When you're beginning, a quiet place and a relaxation tape often help. And remember, a wandering mind is normal when you start out. Just keep bringing your attention back to relaxation.

Deep breathing. Deep breathing from your diaphragm is relaxing. It also exchanges more carbon dioxide for oxygen, to give you more energy. Try to incorporate 20 minutes of deep breathing daily, not just when you're stressed. See "Taking a breather" on page 201.

Progressive muscle relaxation. This technique involves relaxing a series of muscles one at a time. First, raise the tension level in a group of muscles, such as in a leg or an arm, by tightening the muscles and then relaxing them. Concentrate on letting the tension go in each muscle. Then move on to the next muscle group. Be careful, however, not to tense muscles near your pain sites.

Guided imagery. Also known as visualization, this method of relaxation involves lying quietly and picturing yourself in a pleasant and peaceful setting. You experience the setting with all of your senses as if you were actually there. For instance, imagine lying on the beach. Picture the beautiful blue sky, smell the salt water, hear the waves and feel the warm breeze on your skin. The messages your brain receives as you experience these senses help you to relax.

Get SMART

Here are some stress reduction goals that follow the SMART formula:

Goal: Use deep breathing to relax tense muscles
When I want to achieve it: 2 weeks
How I'm going to do it: At least twice a day, practice deep, relaxed diaphragmatic breathing
How I'm going to measure it: In my journal, rate my stress level daily and indicate if deep breathing worked in stressful situations

Goal: Simplify my schedule
When I want to achieve it: 1 month
How I'm going to do it: Delegate some current duties and don't take on any new tasks unless absolutely necessary
How I'm going to measure it: Compare this month's daily planner with next month's to see if next month I have fewer commitments

Chapter 16

Interacting with family and friends

A s trying as your pain is for you, it can be every bit as troubling to your family and friends. They want to help you, but they may not know how. So they say or do things they think are helpful but may only add to your frustration.

Because chronic pain is such a personal experience, it's difficult for family and friends to understand exactly what you're going through. In addition, when pain takes over, communication often suffers. You may not feel like discussing your pain or the problems related to it. And family and friends may hesitate to approach certain topics for fear they'll anger or frustrate you.

You need family and friends to help you deal with your pain and move on with your life. Studies show that people with a solid support system — who have family and friends who care about them — generally:

- Cope better with chronic pain
- Are less likely to become depressed
- Are more independent
- Recover faster from illness
- Live longer

Through your own experiences, you may know what researchers are talking about. You've felt how quickly a cup of coffee with a neighbor has lifted your spirits. You've experienced how a helping hand from a relative has helped you get through a bad day. Being around others can help you forget about your frustrations. However, for family and friends to help you, you need to help them.

Building bridges

Good friends and a supportive family can provide encouraging words, offer gentle but helpful criticisms and lend a hand when you need assistance. Family and friends also help replace sadness with smiles and laughter. In this way, they contribute to your health and well-being.

Making friendships and maintaining family ties seem to come more naturally for some people than for others. But even if you're not an outgoing person, you need social support. If your support system is in need of a little strengthening, try these suggestions:

- Answer phone calls and letters.
- Accept invitations to events, even if it feels awkward at first.
- Don't wait to be invited somewhere. Call someone.
- Set aside past differences and approach your relationships with a clean slate.

- Take part in community organizations, neighborhood events and family gatherings.
- Strike up a conversation with the person next to you at a local gathering. You could be introducing yourself to a new friend.
- Talk about things that other people are interested in. Be an alert listener.

Good relationships require patience, compromise and acceptance. Without these things, the relationship can become a source of stress instead of support. Family and friends need to learn to accept you along with your needs, and you need to accept them along with theirs.

It's true that relationships can sometimes be difficult. Your friends and family may want more of your time and energy than you can spare. But instead of pulling away from those you're close to, educate them about your pain. And allow friends and family members to tell you how your pain has affected them.

This will help those closest to you understand why you may not always be able to do all of the things they ask. It will also help you understand how your pain affects others.

Talking openly and honestly

Discussing your thoughts and feelings can be difficult even in the best of times. With chronic pain, the task doesn't get any easier. Instead of continually telling people what you're going through and how you're feeling, it's often easier to withdraw or say as little as possible.

The problem with this approach is that it can frustrate and alienate your family and friends. They may not know how to interpret your withdrawal and won't know that you're having a bad day unless you tell them. You don't have to go on about your symptoms, but simply saying "I'm having a rough day" or "I need some space" will let them know you need time to yourself.

If you're having difficulty talking with family and friends about your pain,

How does your social network stack up?

A strong support system is associated with better health and a longer life. Check each statement that's true about your relationships. Each statement marks an important link in your social network.

_____ I have friends or family members nearby to help me.
_____ I'm involved in a community or religious organization.
_____ I have at least one friend or relative that I can talk to about almost anything.
_____ I keep in daily contact with other people.

Statements you didn't mark are areas you might work on to improve your support system.

don't give up. Consider these suggestions as you take steps to improve communications.

Express what you're feeling. The only way people can begin to understand what you're thinking or feeling is if you tell them. But do it in a positive manner, not one in which you appear to be whining or accusatory. Negative emotions only increase your chances for a negative response.

For example, if you're frustrated because your friends don't include you in their activities, you might say, "I miss spending time with you on Saturdays, and I sure would like to join you on a walk or bicycling." Your friends may incorrectly assume you can't take part in recreational events. That's why they don't invite you along, not because they don't want to be around you.

Don't lie about your pain. Close family and friends may know not to ask how you're doing every time they see you. But some people won't understand that you may always have some degree of pain. When they inquire how you're doing, don't pretend it doesn't hurt. But don't exaggerate your pain, either. You might respond, "I still have pain, but I'm learning to manage it."

Ask for help when you need it. You were probably taught to cherish your independence, so it may be difficult for you to ask for help. But sometimes you need help. Try asking in a way that explains what's going on. For example: "I've invited friends over for dinner, and it's taking me longer to get the meal prepared than I anticipated. Could you please come over and lend me a hand for a while?"

Say 'thank you' — and mean it. When someone helps you or gives you a heartfelt compliment about progress you're making, say thanks. Don't feel depressed that you needed the help.

Talk about what bugs you. If the flow of communication between you and a family member or friend becomes one-sided, talk about it. Set aside your pride for a while and take the risk of saying exactly how you feel. If that fails to open the channel, don't give up too soon.

If you can't say it out loud, spell it out. Use your journal to express those feelings you have trouble communicating. This not only will buy you time to let these feelings settle but also will give you practice in expressing them when you're ready to discuss them.

How family and friends can help

Chances are your family and friends have asked you what they can do to help you. Perhaps you didn't know what to say, or you felt guilty admitting that you needed any type of special treatment. Or maybe they've decided to help in ways that irritate you. They think they're doing things to make you feel better, but they're not.

When people ask you how they can help, tell them. Here are some suggestions you might pass along:

Don't always talk about my pain. It's easy for friends and family to get caught up in discussing your pain. But that only reminds you of your condition and draws attention to your pain — something you're trying to avoid.

Try not to hover over me. Being overly attentive to someone with persistent pain can actually interfere with rehabilitation. One study found that people with chronic pain who were cared for by an overly attentive spouse reported more pain than when they were observed by someone else. Tell your spouse or partner that you appreciate the concern, but that he or she doesn't need to be your servant. You need to learn to do things for yourself.

Join me in activities. Having friends and family members accompany you for a walk or go with you to support meetings or doctor visits can offer many benefits. Having friends or family members along gives you a chance to talk and share time together. It also gives friends and family members an opportunity to learn more about your need to exercise and stay active.

Don't give up things you enjoy for my sake. Those closest to you may consciously or unconsciously change their lifestyle because of your pain. But that only makes you feel guilty. For example, if you and a friend enjoyed fishing together, don't let your friend sell his tackle just because he thinks you can't fish anymore. Perhaps you can't fish from dawn to dusk as you used to, but you still may be able to fish for a few hours.

Be available to listen to me. Sometimes you simply need someone to listen. A family member or friend who understands that you're not asking them to fix the problem can lend emotional support by just listening to you. This can provide a release valve for your daily stresses. People who feel they have the support of loved ones seem to cope better with their pain and live more active lives.

Take care of yourself. Your pain, and worrying about you, can take a toll on friends and family members. It's important that those you care about take care of their health as well. Just as you need their support, they need yours.

Get SMART

Here are some goals for building friendships and improving communication that follow the SMART formula:

Goal: Spend less time by myself
When I want to achieve it: 2 months
How I'm going to do it: Call my friend Annie at least once a week, join co-workers for gatherings after work, attend social events at church and in the neighborhood
How I'm going to measure it: Keep track in my journal of the hours I spend with others compared with the hours I'm alone

Goal: Talk more openly with family about how I'm feeling
When I want to achieve it: 1 month
How I'm going to do it: Set aside Sunday evenings as family time to talk about how we're feeling and the week ahead, and be honest
How I'm going to measure it: Jot down in my journal how family time went — what worked and what didn't — and if it seems to get easier talking about my feelings

Chapter 17

Caring for yourself

L iving well with chronic pain isn't just about managing the pain. It's about caring for your overall health so that you can enjoy life to its fullest. Getting more physically active, reducing stress and learning to relax were discussed earlier. This chapter focuses on other factors — including sleep, weight and diet, alcohol and smoking, and your spiritual needs — that can help you stay active and productive.

Getting a good night's sleep

Sleep refreshes you. It improves your attitude and gives you energy for physical activity and to fight off fatigue and stress. It also boosts your immune system, reducing your risk of illness.

If you aren't sleeping well, it may be because your pain is keeping you from falling asleep or is waking you up at night. Other factors that can interfere with sleep are:

- Stress
- Stimulant medications
- Anxiety
- Regular use of sleeping pills
- Depression
- Alcohol
- Lack of physical activity
- Poor sleep habits
- Change in your environment

To improve your sleep, it's important to recognize factors that may be contributing to your restless nights.

Stages of sleep

During the night, you cycle from light sleep to deep sleep and back to light sleep. Most people typically experience four to six sleep cycles, moving from one stage to another with each cycle lasting about 90 minutes.

There are two types of sleep — non-rapid eye movement (NREM) sleep and rapid eye movement (REM). Your nightly journey begins as you pass into stage one of NREM sleep, a light sleep. During NREM sleep, your brain activity and body functions slow. Later stages of NREM sleep, called delta sleep or deep sleep, are the most restful. In these stages, brain waves are large and slow, and you're more difficult to awaken.

REM, or dream, sleep occurs about one and a half to two hours after you fall asleep. In this sleep, brain activity increases and your eyes move rapidly behind your closed eyelids, hence the name. Your body, however, typically doesn't move. You do more thinking, in the form or dreaming, in this stage.

Sleep is important, because it restores you mentally, emotionally and physically. Lack of sleep not only affects your energy level, but also your social and mental functioning. Losing sleep can cause difficulty with concentration and increased irritability. Insomnia also may be related to depression.

Strategies to help you sleep better

Before bed, take time to relax. Doing so will help you sleep better. Some of the many activities that promote relaxation include:

- Deep breathing and muscle relaxation techniques
- Taking a warm bath
- Having a light snack
- Reading
- Listening to soothing music
- Writing in your journal

Relaxation helps reduce your pain so that you can fall asleep more easily. It also helps you achieve more restful sleep. Here are other suggestions that may help you sleep better:

Establish regular sleep hours. Go to bed and wake up at the same time each day — even on weekends.

Limit your time in bed. Too much sleep can promote shallow, unrestful sleep. To the contrary, spending too much time in bed also disrupts sleep. Nine out of 10 people with insomnia stay in bed longer than necessary.

Don't try to sleep. The harder you try, the more awake you'll become. Read or watch television until you become drowsy and fall asleep naturally.

Limit bedroom activities. Save your bedroom for sleep and sex. Don't

To nap, or not?

The urge for a midday snooze is built into your body's biological clock. It generally hits between 1 p.m. and 4 p.m., when your body temperature naturally dips slightly. Napping shouldn't be viewed as a substitute for a full night's sleep. You shouldn't nap if you have trouble sleeping at night. However, if you find that a nap refreshes you and doesn't interfere with nighttime sleep, it's OK to take one, provided you:

Keep it short. Thirty minutes is ideal. Naps longer than one to two hours are more likely to interfere with your nighttime sleep.

Take a midafternoon nap. Naps at this time produce a physically invigorating slumber.

Simply rest awhile, if you can't sleep. Lie down and keep your mind on something relaxing.

watch TV or take your work materials to bed.

Watch what you eat. A light snack may help you relax before sleeping. However, avoid heavy meals and fluids or foods that stimulate stomach acid production, which could cause heartburn or irritate your esophagus.

Avoid or limit caffeine, alcohol and nicotine. Caffeine and nicotine can keep you from falling asleep. Alcohol may make you sleepy but it often causes unrestful sleep and frequent awakenings during the night.

Minimize interruptions. Close your bedroom door or create a subtle background noise, such as that from a fan, to muffle other noises. Drink less before you go to bed so that you won't have to get up during night to go to the bathroom.

Get comfy. Make sure you have a bed that's comfortable and keep your bedroom temperature at a comfortably cool level.

Hide the clock. A visible indicator of how long you've been unable to sleep may make you needlessly anxious. Place clocks where they aren't visible or within reach.

Keep active. Regular physical activity helps you sleep more soundly. Try to get at least 30 minutes of physical activity daily, preferably five to six hours before bedtime. Also keep occupied throughout the day. Boredom promotes restless sleep.

Avoid or limit naps. Naps can make it harder to fall asleep at night.

Schedule worry time. Your bedroom is your sanctuary for sleep. Don't take your worries to bed with you. Before you go to bed, take time to address your worries and think of ways you might solve them.

Check your medications. Ask your doctor if your medications might be contributing to your difficulty sleeping. Also check over-the-counter products that you're taking to see if they contain caffeine or other stimulants, such as pseudoephedrine.

What about sleep medications?

If you're having trouble sleeping, your doctor may prescribe a sleep medication until other steps to improve your sleep and control your pain have time to take effect.

The downfall of many prescription and over-the-counter sleep medications is that they often don't allow you to experience all phases of sleep. The drugs can also lose their effectiveness and cause side effects, including dry mouth, next-day drowsiness and physical dependence. Plus, over time, they can actually make it more difficult for you to get restful sleep.

For sleep difficulties associated with chronic pain, antidepressants are often prescribed (see page 92). A side effect of some antidepressants is drowsiness. When taken before bed, they can help you sleep.

Controlling your weight

Maintaining a healthy weight reduces your risk of illnesses such as cardiovascular disease, high blood pressure and diabetes. It's also easier to manage your pain when you're not overweight. That's because excessive weight saps your energy level, increases stress on muscles and joints, and decreases your flexibility.

It's not necessary that you become thin. But losing even a few pounds may help reduce your level of pain, as well as your blood sugar and cholesterol levels.

Is your weight healthy?

Three do-it-yourself evaluations can tell you if your weight is healthy or whether you could benefit from weight loss.

Body mass index. Body mass index (BMI) is a formula that considers your weight and your height in determining whether you have a healthy or unhealthy percentage of total body fat. It's a better measurement of health risks related to your weight than using your bathroom scale or standard height-and-weight tables.

To determine your BMI, locate your height on the chart on the next page and follow it across until you reach the weight nearest yours. Look at the top of the column for the BMI rating. If your weight is less than the weight nearest yours, your BMI may be slightly less. If your weight is greater than the weight nearest yours, your BMI may be slightly greater. A BMI of 18.5 to 24.9 is considered healthy. A BMI of 25 to 29.9 signifies overweight, and a BMI of 30 or more indicates obesity.

Waist circumference. This measurement indicates where most of your body fat is located. People who carry most of their weight around their waists may be referred to as apple-like. Those who carry most of their weight below their waists, around their hips and thighs, may be described as pear-like.

Generally, it's better to have a pear shape than to have an apple shape. That's because fat around your abdomen is associated with a greater risk of cardiovascular and other weight-related diseases.

Body mass index (BMI)

You can determine your body mass index (BMI) by finding your height and weight on this chart. A BMI of 18.5 to 24.9 is considered the healthiest. People with a BMI under 18.5 are considered underweight. People with a BMI between 25 and 29.9 are considered overweight. People with a BMI of 30 or greater are considered obese.

	Healthy		Overweight					Obese				
BMI	**19**	**24**	**25**	**26**	**27**	**28**	**29**	**30**	**35**	**40**	**45**	**50**
Height						Weight in pounds						
4'10"	91	115	119	124	129	134	138	143	167	191	215	239
4'11"	94	119	124	128	133	138	143	148	173	198	222	247
5'0"	97	123	128	133	138	143	148	153	179	204	230	255
5'1"	100	127	132	137	143	148	153	158	185	211	238	264
5'2"	104	131	136	142	147	153	158	164	191	218	246	273
5'3"	107	135	141	146	152	158	163	169	197	225	254	282
5'4"	110	140	145	151	157	163	169	174	204	232	262	291
5'5"	114	144	150	156	162	168	174	180	210	240	270	300
5'6"	118	148	155	161	167	173	179	186	216	247	278	309
5'7"	121	153	159	166	172	178	185	191	223	255	287	319
5'8"	125	158	164	171	177	184	190	197	230	262	295	328
5'9"	128	162	169	176	182	189	196	203	236	270	304	338
5'10"	132	167	174	181	188	195	202	209	243	278	313	348
5'11"	136	172	179	186	193	200	208	215	250	286	322	358
6'0"	140	177	184	191	199	206	213	221	258	294	331	368
6'1"	144	182	189	197	204	212	219	227	265	302	340	378
6'2"	148	186	194	202	210	218	225	233	272	311	350	389
6'3"	152	192	200	208	216	224	232	240	279	319	359	399
6'4"	156	197	205	213	221	230	238	246	287	328	369	410

Note: Asians with a BMI of 23 or higher may have an increased risk of health problems. Source: National Institutes of Health, 1998

You can calculate your exact BMI by using this formula:

$$\left(\frac{\text{Weight in pounds}}{(\text{Height in inches}) \times (\text{Height in inches})} \right) \times 703 = \text{BMI}$$

For example, if you weigh 165 pounds and you're 5 feet 10 inches tall, your BMI is 23.7.

$$\left(\frac{165 \text{ pounds}}{(70 \text{ inches}) \times (70 \text{ inches})} \right) \times 703 = 23.7$$

To determine whether you're carrying too much weight around your abdomen, measure your waist circumference. Find the highest point on each of your hipbones and measure across your abdomen just above those points. A measurement of more than 40 inches (102 centimeters) in men and 35 inches (89 centimeters) in women signifies increased health risks, especially if you have a BMI of 25 or more.

Personal and family history. An evaluation of your medical history, along with that of your family, is equally important in determining whether your weight is healthy. Answer these questions:

- Do you have a health condition, such as arthritis or back pain, that would benefit from weight loss?
- Do you have a family history of a weight-related illness, such as diabetes, high blood pressure or high cholesterol?
- Have you gained considerable weight since high school? Weight gain in adulthood is associated with increased health risks.
- Do you smoke cigarettes, have more than two alcoholic drinks a day or live with considerable stress? In combination with these

behaviors, excess weight can have greater health implications.

Adding up the results. If your BMI shows you aren't overweight, you're not carrying too much weight around your abdomen and you answered no to all of the personal or family history questions, there's probably no health advantage to changing your weight. Your weight is healthy. However, it's important for you to maintain good eating and exercise habits to help keep you from gaining weight.

If your BMI is between 25 and 29.9, your waist circumference exceeds healthy guidelines or you answered yes to at least one personal and family health question, you might benefit from losing a few pounds. Discuss your weight with your doctor during your next visit.

If your BMI is 30 or more, losing weight will improve your overall health and energy level and reduce your risk of future illness.

Losing weight successfully

The best way to lose weight safely and keep it off permanently is through lifestyle changes. There are many products and programs that promise to help you shed pounds, but they aren't always safe or effective. Once you go off the diet, you almost always gain the weight back again. To increase your chances of being successful:

Make a commitment. You must be motivated to lose weight because it's what you want, not what someone else wants you to do. Only you can lose weight. But that doesn't mean you have to do everything alone. Your doctor or a registered dietitian can help you plan how best to lose weight.

Think positively. Don't dwell on what you're giving up to lose weight. Instead, concentrate on what you're gaining. Instead of thinking, "I really miss eating a doughnut for breakfast," tell yourself, "I feel a lot better when I eat whole-wheat toast and cereal in the morning."

Set a realistic goal. Don't aim for a weight that's unrealistic. If you've always been overweight, aim for a weight that will help reduce pressure on your joints and muscles and improve your energy level. Studies show that losing even 10 percent of

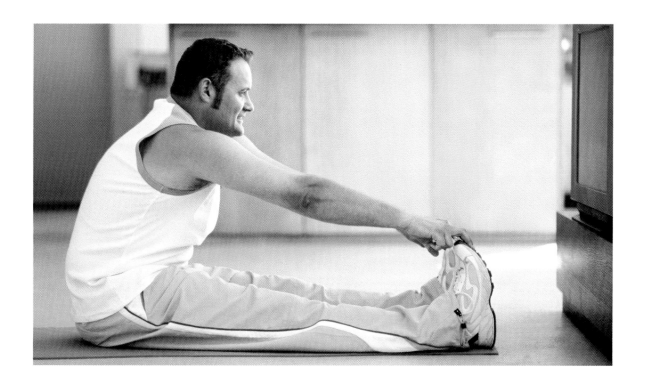

what you weigh can improve your health and sense of well-being. Because weight can fluctuate considerably over the short term due to a variety of factors, your goals should include behaviors that are within your control.

Accept that healthy weight loss is slow and steady. A good weight loss plan generally involves losing no more than 1 to 2 pounds a week. Set weekly or monthly goals that allow you to check off your successes. Reward yourself when you meet a goal.

Know your habits. Ask yourself if you tend to eat when you're bored, angry, tired, anxious, depressed or socially pressured. If you do, try these possible solutions:

- Before eating anything, ask yourself if you really want it.
- Do something to distract yourself from your desire to eat, such as telephone a friend or run an errand.
- If you're feeling stressed or angry, direct that energy constructively. Instead of eating, practice a relaxation technique or take a long, brisk walk.

Don't starve yourself. Many people try to lose weight by eating 1,000 to 1,500 calories a day. Cutting calories to fewer than 1,200 if you're a woman or 1,400 if you're a man doesn't provide enough food to keep you satisfied. When you're hungry, your risk of overeating or eating unhealthy foods is greater. Plus, too few calories promotes temporary loss of fluids and loss of healthy muscle, instead of permanent loss of fat.

Get and stay active. Eating more healthfully will help you lose weight, but adding 30 minutes of moderate activity most days of the week will help increase your rate of weight loss. Physical activity is the most important factor related to long-term weight loss. It promotes loss of body fat and development of muscle. These changes in body composition raise the rate at which you burn calories, making it easier to maintain your weight loss. Only you will know how much you can exercise. Pain may impose limits on the types of exercise you do. However, exercise may also relieve pain and stiffness.

Think lifelong. It's not enough to eat healthy foods and exercise for a few weeks or even several months. As with other strategies for managing your pain, you have to incorporate these new behaviors into your life.

Eating better

Food can't control your pain. But a nutritionally balanced diet can improve the way you feel. In addition to helping you lose weight, eating a variety of foods gives you energy and a sense of well-being.

Experts agree that the best way to increase nutrients in your diet and limit fat and calories is to eat more plant-based foods. Plant foods — fruits, vegetables and foods made from whole grains — contain beneficial vitamins, minerals, fibers and health-enhancing compounds called phytochemicals. By emphasizing plant foods in your diet, you increase consumption of many naturally healthy compounds.

For good health and better success at controlling your weight, eat a healthy balance of these foods each day.

Vegetables. Eat at least four servings of vegetables every day. Vegetables are naturally low in calories, and almost all are fat-free. They provide vitamins, minerals, fiber and phytochemicals.

Fresh vegetables are best, but frozen vegetables are good, too. Most canned vegetables are high in sodium, which is used as a preservative in the canning process. Excessive sodium can increase blood pressure in some people. If you eat canned vegetables, select those indicating that no sodium has been added or the sodium is reduced.

Fruits. You can also eat fruit in unlimited quantities, with the exception of dried fruit and fruit juices, which are high in calories. Try to include at least three servings of fruit daily.

Fruit contains little or no fat, and it provides many beneficial nutrients and phytochemicals. Fresh fruit is generally best. It makes a great snack. If you get the urge to snack between meals or you have a sweet tooth, keep a bowl of fresh fruit nearby. Frozen fruits with no added sugar and fruits canned in water or their own juices are acceptable alternatives.

Carbohydrates. Carbohydrates include grain products, such as cereals, breads, rice and pasta, and starchy vegetables, such as corn, potatoes and some types of squash.

Along with vegetables and fruits, carbohydrates should form the foundation of your daily diet. Whenever possible,

select whole-grain foods over refined products. Whole grains contain bran and germ, which add fiber. Whole grains are also important sources of vitamins and minerals.

Some carbohydrates, such as croissants, crackers and dessert breads, are high in fat and calories. But most plain cereals, breads and pasta are low in fat and calories. It's what you put on these foods — whole milk, cream, or spreads and sauces made from fats, oils or cheese — that adds calories.

Protein and dairy. Protein is an essential nutrient that helps maintain body tissues, such as skin, bone and muscle. Protein is found in a variety of foods, including milk, yogurt, cheese, eggs, meat, poultry, fish and legumes (beans, dried peas and lentils). Most Americans eat far more protein than they need, especially those products that are high in fat and calories, such as meat.

Make sure to include low-fat or fat-free milk or milk products (yogurt and cheese) in your daily diet. Milk, yogurt and cheese are major sources of calcium and vitamin D. Calcium helps keep your bones healthy and reduces your risk of osteoporosis, a disease that reduces bone density and makes your bones brittle. Adequate vitamin D is also important to bone health.

Always try to select fat-free or low-fat varieties of protein, such as poultry (without skin), fish, lean meats, legumes, skim milk and low-fat cheeses.

Fats. A small amount of fat in your diet is necessary to help your body function, but most people consume far more fat than they need. Foods high in fat include products produced mainly from oils, butter, margarine, salad dressing or mayonnaise. An easy way to reduce fat in your diet is to reduce the amount of oil, butter and margarine you add to food when preparing it. Many snack products, such as chips and crackers, also are high in fat.

Healthier fats include those that contain monounsaturated fat, such as olive oil and canola oil. But even these should be eaten sparingly.

Sweets. Sweets such as candy and desserts contain considerable calories, and they offer little in terms of nutrition. Many sweets are also high in fat. You don't have to give up sweets

entirely to eat healthfully, but be smart about your selections and portion sizes. Instead of sugar-sweetened soft drinks, candy bars or pastries, consider healthier choices, such as water, fresh fruit, low-fat frozen yogurt, angel food cake or reduced-calorie cookies.

Limiting alcohol

The best advice about alcohol is that if you drink, do it in moderation (see page 224). And if you're taking medication, it might be best not to drink any alcohol.

Alcohol can increase the potency and side effects of many prescription drugs, including pain relievers and antidepressants. In addition, regularly combining alcohol with over-the-counter pain relievers, including acetaminophen or nonsteroidal anti-inflammatory drugs (NSAIDs), may increase your risk of liver damage.

Using alcohol to help relieve your pain can also lead to dependence and addiction. If you regularly drink more than a moderate amount of alcohol, talk with your doctor about the safest and most successful way to limit alcohol.

What's moderate drinking?

Moderate drinking means no more than one alcoholic drink each day for women and no more than two alcoholic drinks daily for men. One drink equals one 12-ounce (360-milliliter, mL) bottle of beer, one 5-ounce (150-mL) glass of wine or one 1.5-ounce (45-mL) shot glass of 80-proof liquor.

For men and women age 65 and older, moderate drinking is one drink daily. The amount is less for older individuals because they typically process alcohol more slowly.

Quitting smoking

There's no question smoking is dangerous to your health. Tobacco smoke contains more than 4,000 substances that can damage your heart and blood vessels and cause cancer. Smoking also contributes to chronic pain by increasing fatigue and muscle weakness. Carbon monoxide in tobacco smoke replaces oxygen in your red blood cells. Less oxygen means less energy and fewer nutrients for your body tissues.

Breaking tobacco's grip

Some people can simply stop and never smoke again. For others, quitting takes several tries and various approaches. Don't let one failed attempt to quit keep you from trying again. You can learn from previous attempts, increasing your chances for being successful in the future. Follow these steps:

Do your homework. That way you'll know what to expect. You may experience physical withdrawal symptoms for at least 10 days. Common symptoms include irritability, anxiety and loss of concentration. Afterward, you may still have the urge to light up in familiar smoking situations, such as after a meal or while driving. These urges are generally very brief, but they can be very strong.

By knowing what to expect and having alternative activities planned, you'll be better prepared to handle the urges. These activities might include chewing gum after a meal or snacking on carrot sticks when you need to keep your hands busy.

Set a stop date. For some people, quitting cold turkey works better than cutting down gradually. Carefully select a date to quit smoking. Many smokers choose to quit during vacation or while on a trip when they're away from their usual routines and smoking situations. One reason is that your routine often changes while on vacation. It's easier to break free of smoking rituals when you're away than when you're at work or home.

Tell others about your decision. Having the support of family, friends and co-workers can help you reach your goal more quickly. However, many smokers keep their plans to quit a secret because they don't want to look like a failure if they go back to smoking. Many people try three or more times before they're successful, so don't give up.

Start changing your routine. Before your stop date, cut down on the number of places you smoke. For instance, stop smoking in your car, and smoke in only one room of the house or outside. This approach will help reduce your smoking urges so that you can be more comfortable in those places without smoking.

Talk with your doctor about medications. Nicotine is a highly addictive substance. Withdrawal from nicotine can cause irritability, anxiety and difficulty concentrating. Medications are available that can help lessen withdrawal symptoms and increase your chances of being successful.

Take it one day at a time. On your stop day, quit completely. Each day, focus your attention on remaining tobacco-free.

Avoid smoking situations. Leave the table right after meals if this is the time you used to light up. If you smoked

Medications to help you stop smoking

Most people use at least one medication when they try to stop smoking, but many find that a combination of medications is the most comfortable and effective approach. Use them according to your doctor's instructions or, in the case of over-the-counter (OTC) medications, according to instructions on the label.

Nicotine replacement products deliver small doses of nicotine to help relieve withdrawal symptoms but don't keep a smoker addicted to the substance. These products are considered temporary aids — usually for several weeks and at most several months. Consult your doctor about tapering off these medications.

Nicotine patches. Similar to an adhesive bandage, a nicotine patch is placed on your skin and gradually releases nicotine into your body. It's an over-the-counter product and comes in different sizes — the larger the patch, the more nicotine delivered. To minimize skin irritation, rotate the site of the patch and apply an OTC cortisone cream.

Nicotine gum. This OTC product isn't intended to be chewed like normal gum. Bite into the nicotine gum a few times, then "park" it between your cheek and gum and leave it there. The lining of your mouth absorbs the nicotine that the gum releases. Two doses are available — 2 milligrams (mg) and 4 mg. Chew enough gum to relieve symptoms.

Nicotine lozenges. The nicotine lozenge was introduced as a nonprescription product in 2002. It looks like a hard candy and releases nicotine as it slowly dissolves in the mouth. Doses are available in 2-mg and 4-mg amounts — the 4-mg lozenge is used by heavier smokers.

Nicotine nasal spray. You spray this product into your nose with a bottle dispenser. The nicotine is absorbed into your bloodstream through the lining of your nose, providing a quicker response to nicotine cravings than the other products provide. It's intended mainly for when you need immediate relief from withdrawal symptoms, and often used with nicotine patch therapy or with bupropion medication. The product is available only by prescription.

Nicotine inhaler. This device looks like a plastic cigarette that you put to your mouth and puff on, releasing a nicotine vapor into your mouth. Although it's called an inhaler, it doesn't deliver nicotine to the lungs. This product is available only by prescription and the dose is individualized. Using an inhaler also helps smokers who miss the hand-to-mouth ritual that's part of smoking a cigarette.

Non-nicotine medications. Bupropion (Zyban) is a non-addicting, non-nicotine medication approved by the Food and Drug Administration (FDA) as a stop-smoking aid. It's not clear exactly how the drug works. One theory is that bupropion stimulates dopamine, a brain chemical that causes a feel-good response similar to that produced by nicotine and other addictive drugs. Bupropion is available only by prescription.

Varenicline (Chantix) is the most recent prescription drug approved by the FDA to stop smoking. This medication stimulates the same brain receptors that are usually activated by the nicotine in tobacco products. Chantix also blocks some of the pleasure you get from smoking, making smoking less rewarding.

while using the telephone, avoid long phone conversations or talk while doing other things. If you had a favorite smoking chair, avoid it.

You'll soon be able to anticipate when the urge to smoke will hit you. Before it hits, start doing something that makes smoking inconvenient, such as washing your car or doing relaxation exercises. Your smoking behavior is deeply ingrained and automatic. You need to anticipate your reflex behavior and plan alternatives.

Time each urge. Check your watch when a smoking urge hits. Most are short. Once you realize this, it's easier to resist. Tell yourself, "I can make it another few minutes and then the urge will pass."

Expressing your sexuality

Sexuality is a natural and healthy part of living, and a part of your identity as a man or woman. It involves the timeless desire for both physical and emotional intimacy. Sexuality can be expressed through shared interests, companionship or holding hands, as well as physical contact, including sexual intercourse.

When chronic pain invades your life, the pleasures of sexuality often disappear. You may not feel like socializing, sharing your thoughts and feelings or having close contact. Perhaps you feel your pain has made you less desirable to your partner. Your sleeping arrangement may even have changed. Some people sleep in a spare bedroom or a lounger because they have difficulty getting comfortable or they don't want to keep their partner awake.

In spite of your pain, you can have a healthy and satisfying sexual relationship. It begins with honest communication. You and your partner need to talk about how you feel, what you miss and what you would like from your relationship. You also need to be creative and willing to make changes. That could be as basic as buying a new mattress or a bigger bed so that you don't have to sleep apart, or exploring different ways to express your sexuality.

In all partnerships it takes effort to maintain what's good and to correct what isn't. A healthy sexual relationship can positively affect all aspects of your life, including your physical health, self-esteem, productivity and other relationships.

Becoming more intimate

Start slowly. Before concentrating on improving your sexual relationship, spend time talking. Get to know one another again. Also look for ways to rekindle your romance. Go on a date, plan a picnic, send flowers or exchange personal gifts.

Remind yourself that problems are also opportunities. In your efforts to become more intimate you may discover something about your partner you otherwise might have missed. The relationship you recover may be even better than the one you had before your pain.

Fears about resuming sexual intercourse

You or your partner may have unspoken fears regarding sexual contact and, because of this, may avoid intimate encounters. Delaying intimacy only increases the anxiety surrounding sexual intercourse. Talking openly with your partner about your fears often can help ease them.

Fear of increased pain. It's natural to want to avoid additional pain. And it's common to worry that sexual intercourse will cause you physical pain, especially if your pain is centered in your back, abdomen or pelvis.

Experimenting with different positions and other ways to satisfy your and your partner's sexual needs can help the two of you enjoy intimate encounters (see "Making love creatively" on page 230). Relaxation exercises before and after intercourse also may help reduce fears and manage pain.

Fear of partner rejection. This is a common feeling. You may wonder if your partner is less attracted to you because of your pain. The longer you have these fears, the more difficult it may be to overcome them. Talk openly with your partner about your feelings and fears and encourage your partner to do the same.

Fear of failure to perform. If you're having difficulty becoming sexually aroused, maintaining an erection or achieving an orgasm, talk with your doctor. Your pain itself, depression, concern over your physical appearance, alcohol and medications all can affect your sexual performance.

In addition, many medications, including antidepressants, sedatives and opioids, can reduce your sexual ability, including making you impotent. If you suspect a medication may be affecting your sexual performance, don't stop

Making love creatively

Sexual intercourse is just one way to satisfy your need for human closeness. Intimacy can be expressed in many different ways.

Touch. Exploring your partner's body through touch is an exciting way to express your sexual feelings. This can include cuddling, fondling, stroking, massaging and kissing. Touch in any form increases feelings of intimacy.

Self-stimulation. Masturbation is a normal and healthy way to fulfill your sexual needs. One partner may use masturbation during mutual sexual activity if the other partner is unable to be very active.

Timing. A change in the time of day you have sexual intercourse may improve your lovemaking. Many people often have higher pain levels in the evening. If this is true for you, you and your partner might try intercourse in the morning or afternoon.

Experiment with different positions. Lie side by side, kneel or sit. There are many books and brochures available that describe different ways to have intercourse.

Vibrators and lubricants. A vibrator can add pleasure without physical exertion. If lack of natural lubrication is a problem, over-the-counter lubricants can prevent pain associated with vaginal dryness.

taking the drug without first consulting your doctor.

Sometimes, failure to perform is simply a result of stress and anxiety. Patience and understanding can often help you overcome the problem.

Addressing your spiritual needs

The role of spirituality is an important aspect of a person's well-being that's often overlooked. People tend to use the term *spirituality* interchangeably with *religion*. However, the terms aren't necessarily synonymous. Spirituality is as much connected with the spirit and the soul as it is with any specific belief or form of worship. Spirituality is about meaning, values and purpose in life.

Religion may be one way of expressing spirituality, but it's not the only way. For some people, spirituality is feeling in tune with nature and the universe. For still others, spirituality is expressed through music, meditation or art.

For some people, addressing their spiritual needs brings inner peace and added strength to deal with their pain and stress.

Spirituality and healing

Numerous studies have attempted to measure the effect of spirituality on illness and recovery. In reviewing many of these studies, researchers at Georgetown University School of Medicine found at least 80 percent of the studies suggest spiritual beliefs provide health benefits. People who consider themselves to be spiritual generally live longer, recover from illness more quickly, suffer less depression and addiction, and cope better with serious disease.

No one knows exactly how spirituality affects health. Some experts attribute the healing effect of spirituality to hope, which is known to benefit your immune system. Others liken spiritual acts to meditation, and still others point to the social connectedness spirituality provides.

It's important to remember that although spirituality is associated with healing, it isn't a cure. Spirituality can help you live life more fully despite your symptoms, but it won't cure your pain.

Getting through bad days

Everyone has a bad day now and then. Holidays can be difficult. Then there's bill time, or an unpredicted 10-inch snowfall. A visit from relatives also may qualify.

Whatever the reason for your bad day, you can get through it. One of the best ways to minimize the disruptiveness of a tough day and quickly get back to your usual activities is to plan for it. And the time to plan is when you're having a good day — not a bad one. On a bad day, it may not be easy to think of ways to cope with the problem at hand. In fact, it can be challenging to concentrate on much of anything except the day's souring effect.

Here's how to plan ahead for a difficult day:

Know your warning signs. Do you get a warning sign that a bad day is beginning, such as a headache, excessive fatigue or onset of the blues?

Identify sources of your difficult days. Knowing the most common reasons for your difficult days can help you better prepare for them. Think about some recent bad days. Was there a reason for your increased pain? Could it be from too much stress, overdoing it on the weekends, traveling for work, or getting a visit from a particular friend or relative?

Develop a game plan. When you know a difficult day is coming or you get a warning sign, you often can lessen the negative effects by structuring the day with activities and diversions. Having a written plan can help. Your game plan may include some of the following strategies:

- Maintain a normal schedule. A difficult day is not a time to overdo it — or to do nothing. Lying around won't help your pain improve or the day go by any faster.
- Get out of the house. When you're hurting, it's natural to want to be alone and tend your wounds. But this only gives you more opportunity to think about your pain. Go shopping or visit a friend who can keep you occupied. But steer your conversations away from your pain.
- Seek other diversions. Read something enjoyable. Watch a funny movie or call a friend who has a good sense of humor.

- Try to relax. On a difficult day, spend more time relaxing.
- Keep away from medication. If you've weaned yourself from medication, don't let a bad day tempt you into taking it again. Remind yourself that it's only a temporary solution and that you're better off without it. If you're taking medication, don't change the dose in an attempt to reduce the pain. You only increase your risk of side effects, and the increased dose may not help your pain.
- Say, "This will pass." Because it will.

10 ways to maintain your gains

To stay in control of your pain, regularly use the pain management strategies outlined in this book — daily exercise, moderation skills, relaxation techniques and positive thinking strategies. The more you use them, the more beneficial they'll become. Here are some other suggestions to help you maintain your progress and avoid relapses.

1. Don't forget your goals

Select your areas of greatest concern, then set some specific, measurable and realistic goals to help you deal with those issues. You might be worried, for example, that you'll slip back into your old pain behaviors, such as moaning, complaining or limping. Or maybe you're concerned about keeping up your exercise program. Create a list and check off each goal you reach. To strengthen your motivation, periodically review your checklist.

2. Pull out the contract

Some people find that making a personal commitment to improving their lives and managing their pain helps them follow through with their plans. More than just a goal, a contract becomes a pledge, like other binding agreements you've made throughout your life. If you have a contract, put it where you can see it.

3. Monitor your progress

Keeping track of your accomplishments helps motivate you to continue to strive for your goals. Use charts or some other method to display your progress.

4. Plan your day

When you specifically schedule time for something you want to do — such as exercising or going to a movie — you're more likely to do it. Also use to-do lists or notes marked on a calendar as a way to remind you of your priorities.

5. Keep it positive

Look around your house and get rid of things that might lure you back into unhealthy habits. For example, is your bed still sitting in the living room to avoid having to walk upstairs to your bedroom? Are the drapes pulled to keep your rooms dark? Make your house feel

What about support groups?

Support groups can provide a depth of help and advice that you might not find anywhere else. That's because they put you face to face with people who share many of the symptoms and feelings that you do. But not all support groups are the same. Some are mostly educational and feature discussions led by informed guest speakers, while others are more social and unstructured with meetings becoming a time to visit.

What support groups offer

Benefits of support groups may include:

A sense of belonging, of fitting in. There's a special bond between people whose lives have been disrupted by the same problem. Once you experience how others accept you just as you are, you begin to feel more accepting of yourself.

People who understand what you're going through. Family, friends and doctors can sympathize with your problems, but they often can't empathize because they haven't experienced what you have. Support group members generally know what you're feeling and experiencing.

like a home, not a hospital. When you walk around your house, you want to see evidence of a person who lives a happy and active life.

6. Say, 'yes'

Accept help from others. It doesn't mean that you're failing. The fact is, you need support from others to keep you on track and to help you during difficult days. People who have supportive people around to help them often fare better than do those who don't have support. In addition to asking for support from family and friends, you might consider joining a chronic pain support group.

Exchange of advice. When group members talk, they speak with first hand experience. They can inform you about helpful coping techniques.

Opportunity to make new friends. A group member may become a listener when you need to talk or a companion to exercise with.

When support groups aren't the answer

To gain the most benefit from a support group, you have to be willing to share your thoughts and feelings. You must also be willing to learn about and help others. People who are severely depressed and don't want to talk or who have poor social skills are generally less likely to benefit from support groups.

In addition, not all support groups are beneficial. You want to be in a group where the mood is upbeat and the message is positive. Group meetings that aren't carefully monitored can become settings in which to vent and share only negative feelings that feed on themselves. That isn't the type of group that you want to be associated with.

7. Team up with your doctor

If you're having difficulty, make an appointment to see your doctor. Your doctor, or another health care professional, can be one of your biggest advocates. Keep him or her updated on your progress and obstacles you may encounter. He or she can often help you overcome those obstacles.

8. Talk yourself up

List as many positive statements about yourself as you can and say them to yourself when you're feeling discouraged or in danger of slipping back into some of your old patterns of unhealthy behavior. If you do have a relapse, accept that it happens and move on again, positively.

9. Prepare for challenges

Make a list of situations that could disrupt the positive changes you've made. Prepare a response plan that you can use when needed.

Perhaps you've been walking for 30 minutes each day, but you know the weather will soon be changing and you don't like being outside in the snow or cold. How do you still fit in your walk? One option might be to walk indoors at a nearby mall. Or perhaps a local school allows indoor walking during certain hours. You might also consider buying a treadmill.

Another example might be a change at work. You know that your job is going to change and that you'll be taking on new responsibilities. That worries you. One way you might make the transition easier is by developing a list ahead of time. Write down all of the new things you'll need to learn. Prioritize the list and decide what steps you need to take to learn each task. Knowing ahead of time exactly what you need to do and how you're going to do it can make the transition less stressful.

10. Reward yourself

Rewards are a great way to reinforce positive change. When you reach a goal or successfully execute one of your pain strategies, treat yourself to something enjoyable.

Additional resources

Contact these organizations for more information about chronic pain or associated conditions. Some groups offer free printed materials or videos. Others have publications or videos you can purchase.

**American Academy of
Craniofacial Pain**
1901 N. Roselle Road, Suite 920
Schaumburg, IL 60195-3187
888-705-1434
www.aacfp.org

American Academy of Orofacial Pain
19 Mantua Road
Mount Royal, NJ 08061
856-423-3629
www.aaop.org

American Academy of Pain Medicine
4700 W. Lake Ave.
Glenview, IL 60025
847-375-4731
www.painmed.org

American Chronic Pain Association
P.O. Box 850
Rocklin, CA 95677
800-533-3231
www.theacpa.org

American Headache Society
19 Mantua Road
Mount Royal, NJ 08061
856-423-0043
www.americanheadachesociety.org

**American Headache Society
Committee for Headache Education**
19 Mantua Road
Mount Royal, NJ 08061
856-423-0258
www.achenet.org

American Pain Foundation
201 N. Charles St.
Suite 710
Baltimore, MD 21201-4111
888-615-7246
www.painfoundation.org

American Pain Society
4700 W. Lake Ave.
Glenview, IL 60025
847-375-4715
www.ampainsoc.org

Arthritis Foundation
P.O. Box 7669
Atlanta, GA 30357-0669
800-283-7800
www.arthritis.org

Endometriosis Association
8585 N. 76th Place
Milwaukee, WI 53223
414-355-2200
www.endometriosisassn.org

Fibromyalgia Network
P.O. Box 31750
Tucson, AZ 85751
800-853-2929
www.fmnetnews.com

International Association for the Study of Pain
111 Queen Anne Ave. N.
Suite 501
Seattle, WA 98109-4955
206-283-0311
www.iasp-pain.org

International Foundation for Functional Gastrointestinal Disorders
P.O. Box 170864
Milwaukee, WI 53217-8076
888-964-2001 or 414-964-1799
www.iffgd.org

Interstitial Cystitis Association
110 N. Washington St.
Suite 340
Rockville, MD 20850
301-610-5300
www.ichelp.org

Mayo Clinic Health Solutions
www.MayoClinic.com

National Center for Complementary and Alternative Medicine
9000 Rockville Pike
Bethesda, MD 20892
888-644-6226
nccam.nih.gov

National Chronic Pain Outreach Association
P.O. Box 274
Millboro, VA 24460
www.chronicpain.org

National Headache Foundation
820 N. Orleans
Suite 217
Chicago, IL 60610
888-643-5552
www.headaches.org

National Pain Foundation
300 E. Hampden Ave.
Suite 100
Englewood, CO 80113
www.nationalpainfoundation.org

Neuropathy Association
60 E. 42nd St.
Suite 942
New York, NY 10165
212-692-0662
www.neuropathy.org

Reflex Sympathetic Dystrophy Syndrome Association
P.O. Box 502
Milford, CT 06460
877-662-7737
www.rsds.org

TMJ Association Ltd.
P.O. Box 26770
Milwaukee, WI 53226-0770
262-432-0350
www.tmj.org

Trigeminal Neuralgia Association
925 56th Terrace N.W.
Suite C
Gainesville, FL 32605-6402
800-923-3608
www.fpa-support.org

Glossary

A

addiction. An illness in which a person seeks and consumes a substance, such as alcohol, tobacco or a drug, despite the fact that it causes harm.

aerobic exercise. Aerobic means "with oxygen." In reference to exercise, the term refers to the intensity and duration of activity and the energy fuel being used.

allodynia (al-o-DIN-e-uh). An altered sensation in which normally nonpainful events are felt as pain.

analgesic (an-ul-JE-zik). A medication or agent that reduces pain.

anesthetic. A substance used to abolish sensation.

anticonvulsant. A drug used to prevent seizures, which also can be useful for treating pain.

autonomic nervous system. The portion of the nervous system that regulates involuntary body functions, including those of the heart and intestine. Controls blood flow, digestion and temperature regulation.

B

bursa. A fluid-containing sac near or involving a joint or bony prominence that reduces friction between a tendon and a bone, or between a bone and skin during movement.

C

celiac plexus (SE-le-ak PLEK-sus). A network of nerve fibers in the abdomen that's controlled by the autonomic nervous system. This group of nerves also conducts pain sensation from the abdominal organs, such as the liver, spleen, stomach and pancreas.

corticosteroids. Anti-inflammatory drugs created from or based on a naturally occurring hormone (cortisone) produced by the cortex of the adrenal glands.

cortisone. A naturally occurring hormone produced by the cortex of the adrenal glands. It decreases inflammation.

COX-2 inhibitor. A nonsteroidal anti-inflammatory drug (NSAID) that specifically inhibits an enzyme known as cyclooxygenase-2 (COX-2). These drugs are used to treat pain and may be less likely to cause gastrointestinal bleeding than other NSAIDs.

D

dysthesia. An unpleasant, abnormal sensation, often described as burning or crawling.

E

endorphins. Naturally occurring molecules made up of amino acids. Endorphins stop pain messages by attaching to certain receptors in the brain and spinal cord — the same receptors that respond to morphine.

enkephalins (en-KEF-uh-lins). Naturally occurring molecules in the brain. Enkephalins attach to special receptors in your brain and spinal cord to stop pain messages. They also affect other functions within the brain and nervous system.

epidural anesthesia. A procedure used to provide anesthesia during labor and some surgery. Medication is given through a catheter placed in the back. Also called an epidural block.

ergonomics. The science of designing the job to fit the worker, rather than physically forcing the worker's body to fit the job.

F

facet (FAS-ut) joint. A joint between two adjacent vertebrae. Each vertebra is connected at the intervertebral disk in the front and the two facet joints in the back.

field block injection. A procedure used to relax a muscle or to reduce muscle pain and inflammation. The targeted muscle is injected with a local anesthetic and corticosteroid. Also called trigger point injection.

frontal cortex. The portion of the brain that's involved with reasoning, planning, abstract thought and other complex cognitive functions in addition to motor function.

H

hyperalgesia. Abnormally increased pain sensation.

I

inflammation. The protective response of body tissues to irritation or injury. Inflammation may be acute or chronic. Signs and symptoms are redness, heat, swelling and pain, often accompanied by loss of function.

intraspinal. Within or into the vertebral column, which contains the spinal cord and cerebrospinal fluid.

L

limbic system. The portion of the brain that produces emotions.

local anesthetic. A medication that blocks electrical signals in nerves. It eliminates pain in a specific part of the body and causes intended, temporary paralysis.

M

myofascial pain. Pain and tenderness in the muscles and adjacent fibrous tissues (fascia).

N

narcotics. A group of drugs that help relieve pain by blocking or interfering with transmission of pain messages to the brain. Also referred to as opioids.

nerve block. A local anesthetic that is injected around a nerve, preventing pain messages traveling along that nerve pathway from reaching the brain. Used most often to relieve pain for a short period, such as during a surgery.

neuralgia. Pain that extends along one or more nerve pathways.

neurobiology. A branch of biology that is concerned with the anatomy and physiology of the nervous system.

neurolytic. A substance or procedure that destroys nerves.

neuromodulation. Electrical stimulation of a peripheral nerve, the spinal cord or the brain for relief of pain. It may be done transcutaneously or with an implanted nerve stimulator.

neuropathic pain. Pain that originates from a damaged nerve or nervous system.

neurotransmitters. Chemicals in the brain, such as acetylcholine, serotonin and norepinephrine, that facilitate communication between nerve cells (neurons).

nociceptors (no-sih-SEP-turs). Nerve endings attached to peripheral nerves that detect potential or actual tissue damage. They sense unpleasant situations such as extreme heat, cold or pressure.

nonsteroidal anti-inflammatory drugs (NSAIDs). Medications used to reduce inflammation that aren't corticosteroid based.

O

occupational therapist. A skilled professional who helps people return to ordinary tasks around home and at work by way of lifestyle adaptations and occasionally with the aid of assistive devices.

P

pain behaviors. Responses to pain that include talking about pain, rubbing or protecting an affected part of the body, or avoiding routine activities because of pain.

pain scale. A system of rating pain. Often based on a scale of 0 to 10, with 0 being no pain and 10 being the worst pain imaginable.

pain threshold. The point at which pain is noticeable.

pain tolerance level. The peak amount of pain that a person can endure.

palliative care. Care given to people with chronic, often life-threatening illnesses. Care generally focuses on relieving pain or stopping nausea, enhancing quality of life and psychosocial needs.

patient controlled analgesia (PCA). A system that allows people to control the amount of pain medication they receive. The person pushes a button and a machine delivers a dose of pain medicine into the bloodstream through a vein.

peripheral nerves. Nerves that run from your spinal cord to all other parts of your body. Peripheral nerves transmit messages from the spinal cord and brain to and from other parts of your body, and send sensory signals back to the spinal cord and brain.

phantom pain. Pain or discomfort following amputation that feels as if it comes from the missing limb.

physiatrist. A doctor who specializes in physical medicine and rehabilitation. A physiatrist evaluates and recommends treatments that restore function in people with chronic disease.

physical dependence. The physical condition in which rapid discontinuation of a substance, such as alcohol, tobacco or a drug, causes a withdrawal reaction.

physical therapist. A trained professional who teaches exercises and other physical activities to aid in rehabilitation and maximize physical ability with less pain.

R

rebound pain. When regular use of a pain medication makes a person's pain worse instead of better.

receptors. Located on the outer side of a receiving nerve cell, receptors bind the neurotransmitter to the receiving nerve cell and change the activity of this cell.

reflex sympathetic dystrophy (RSD). A chronic, painful condition that usually affects an arm or leg. Signs and symptoms include intense burning or aching pain along with swelling, sweating and hypersensitivity of the area.

regional anesthesia. Medications used to block pain in a certain region of the body without altering consciousness.

S

sciatica. Achiness that may include tingling, numbness or muscle weakness along the sciatic nerve. This major nerve runs through the buttock muscles into the back of the thigh and divides into two nerves behind the knee that run down into the foot.

selective serotonin reuptake inhibitors (SSRIs). Medications used to relieve depression. May work by increasing the availability of a brain chemical (serotonin) that helps to regulate mood.

serotonin (ser-oh-TOE-nin). A brain chemical (neurotransmitter) that helps to regulate your mood. A lack of it may lead to depression.

somatosensory cortex. A part of the brain responsible for processing stimulation coming from the skin, body wall, muscles, bones, tendons and joints. It plays a part in determining pain intensity.

spinal nerve block. A procedure that's used to relieve pain affecting a broad area, such as the abdomen or the legs. A local anesthetic is injected in or near the spinal column, preventing pain messages traveling along that nerve pathway from reaching the brain.

stellate ganglion block. A procedure designed to relieve pain caused by overactivity of the sympathetic nervous system in the upper extremities, the head or the neck. A local anesthetic is injected into the front of the neck to block sympathetic nerves without blocking sensory pathways.

sympathetic block. An injection of an anesthetic to relieve pain resulting from abnormal activity of the sympathetic nervous system. The sympathetic nerves control circulation and perspiration and are part of your autonomic nervous system.

syndrome. A collection of symptoms that characterize a specific disease or condition.

T

thalamus. A portion of the brain that relays impulses from the sensory nerves. Sensory nerves enable people to feel objects that they touch, and they allow people to feel pain.

tolerance. The point at which a person adapts to a specific substance, so larger amounts of the medication or a new medication is needed to achieve the same results.

topical agents. Medications that are applied to the skin rather than ingested or injected. They can come in the form of a cream or a gel. Also called ointments.

transdermal. Entering via the skin, such as a medicated cream being absorbed through the skin.

tricyclic antidepressants. A group of drugs used to relieve symptoms of depression. These drugs may also help relieve pain.

trigger points. Places on the body where muscles and adjacent fibrous tissue (fascia) are sensitive to touch. These areas are generally in the upper and lower back muscles, but they may occur elsewhere.

W

withdrawal. The physical or psychological state experienced when certain substances or medications are discontinued rapidly.

Index

A

abdominal exercises, 159–160
acceptance, 183
acetaminophen, 76
acupuncture/acupressure, 134–135
acute pain
　　back, 34
　　chronic pain vs., 27–28
　　defined, 27
　　See also chronic pain; pain
aerobic exercises, 156–158
aggressive behavior, 191
alcohol
　　limiting use, 223
　　moderate use, 224
　　side effects, 223
　　in sleep loss, 62
allergies, medication, 73
alternative medicine. *See* complementary and
　　　　alternative medicine
analgesics. *See* simple pain relievers
anesthesiologists, 112
anesthetics. *See* local anesthetics
anger, 55–56, 182
　　identification, 188
　　managing, 188–189
　　release valves, 189
　　symptoms, 189
　　triggers, 188–189
　　See also emotions
antidepressants
　　sleep and, 92–93
　　tricyclic, 86–88
　　See also depression
anti-inflammatory medications, 94
anti-seizure medications, 88–90
　　defined, 88
　　side effects, 88–90
　　types of, 88
anxiety
　　hypnotherapy for, 137
　　managing, 187–188
　　medications, 90–92, 188
anxiolytics, 92
aromatherapy, 129

B

back exercises, 160
back pain, 34–36
　　acute, 34
　　herniated disk, 35–36
　　muscle strain/spasm, 34
　　sciatica, 35
　　See also chronic pain
baclofen, 108
bad days, getting through, 234–235
balance
　　body movement, 177–179
　　breathing and, 176
　　daily habits, 174–176
　　finding, 167–180
　　illustrated, 168
　　moderation, 173–174
　　organization, 173
　　SMART goals, 180
　　time management, 169–170
behavioral cycle
　　decrease in activity stage, 52–53
　　family, 59
　　illustrated, 52, 195
　　increase in activity stage, 53
　　loss of strength stage, 53
　　more pain, less activity stage, 53
　　withdrawal and isolation stage, 53–55
　　See also cycles
behaviors
　　aggressive, 191
　　assertive, 190–193
　　dealing with, 181–196
　　expectations, 190
　　observing, 191–192

arthritis, 31–34
　　defined, 31
　　osteoarthritis, 32–33
　　rheumatoid, 33–34
aspirin, 77
assertive behavior, 190–193
　　defined, 191
　　steps for, 191–193
autonomic nerves, 20

behaviors *continued*
    passive, 191
    responding to, 194
    self-esteem and, 193–194
    SMART goals, 192
    See also emotions
benzocaine, 84
benzodiazepines, 93
biofeedback, 136
body language, 193
body mass index (BMI), 216, 217, 218
body movement, 177–179
    kneeling, 178–179
    lifting, 179
    long-handled tool use, 179
    pulling, 178
    pushing, 178
    reaching, 177–178
Botox injections, 101
brain
    frontal cortex, 24
    limbic system, 24
    pain messages and, 23–24
    in pain response, 24
    somatosensory cortex, 24
breathing
    holding breath and, 176
    for relaxation, 203
    in stress reduction, 201
bupropion, 227
burning mouth syndrome, 41
bursa injections, 100–101
buspirone, 92

C

capsaicin, 85
carpal tunnel syndrome, 44–45
celiac plexus block injections, 104
Chantix, 227
chest and arm exercises, 161
chiropractic, 130–131
chondroitin, 128
chronic pain
    acute pain vs., 27–28
    causes, 28–29
    challenges, 30–31
    characteristics, 27–28
    costs of, 61–68
    cycles, 51–60
    defined, 27
    living well with, 30
    managing, 17–18
    sensations, 27
    sensitization, 29–30
    treating, 16–17

    understanding, 16
    unknown causes, 49–50
chronic pain types, 31–50
    arthritis, 31–34
    back pain, 34–36
    complex regional pain syndrome (CRPS), 36
    fibromyalgia, 37
    headache, 37–40
    IBS, 40–41
    mouth, jaw and face, 41–43
    neck pain, 43
    overuse strain injuries, 44–45
    peripheral neuropathy, 48–49
    postherpetic neuralgia, 49
communication
    with family and friends, 207–208
    about medications, 76
    pain, 54
    in relationships, 66–67
    SMART goals, 210
complementary and alternative medicine, 123–140
    caution, 125
    defined, 123–124
    energy therapies, 133–135
    hands-on therapies, 129–133
    herbs and supplements, 126–128
    hypnosis, 136–137
    magnet therapy, 135
    mind-body therapies, 135–140
    strategies, 124–126
complex regional pain syndrome (CRPS), 36
contracts, 235
control, staying in, 233–238
counterirritant products, 85
COX-2 inhibitors, 77–79
cycles, 51–60
    behavioral, 52–55, 195
    breaking, 60
    emotional, 55–58, 196
    family responses, 58–60

D

daily habits, 174–176
    around house, 175–176
    dressing, 175
    kitchen, 175
    outdoors, 176
daily planner, 171–172
denial, 182
depression, 64–65, 182
    causes, 64–65
    chronic pain and, 64–65, 183
    dealing with, 183–187
    defined, 183
    in emotional cycle, 58

medications, 90–92
pain rehabilitation programs and, 120
symptoms, 64, 183
treatment, 65, 187
See also emotions
devil's claw, 126–128
diet
    carbohydrates, 222
    fats, 223
    fruits, 222
    improving, 221–223
    migraines and, 39
    protein and dairy, 222–223
    sleep and, 214
    sweets, 223
    vegetables, 221–222
    See also lifestyle
discogram, 104
doctors
    selecting, 150
    teaming up with, 238
    See also pain specialists
duloxetine, 88

E

elbow exercises, 153–154
emotional cycle, 55–58
    anger and frustration stage, 55–56
    family, 59
    fear and concern stage, 55
    guilt and withdrawal stage, 56–57
    hope and promise stage, 55
    illustrated, 196
    renewed hope, followed by depression
        stage, 58
    See also cycles
emotional response, 24, 26
emotional upheaval, 63–64
emotions
    associated with grieving, 182–183
    dealing with, 181–196
    expectations, 190
    expressing, 208
    family, 60
    pain and, 63–64
    responding to, 194
    self-esteem and, 193–194
    SMART goals, 192
    See also specific emotions
endometriosis, 45
endorphins, 25
energy therapies, 133–135
enkephalins, 25
epidural injections, 102
exercise(s)

aerobic, 156–158
before starting, 152
chronic pain and, 151
flexibility, 153–154
goals, 163
misconception, 151
plan, 163–165
posture and, 162
range-of-motion, 153
SMART formula, 164
strengthening, 158–162
in stress management, 200
stretching, 154–156
tips, 165–166
expectations
    changing, 190
    pain rehabilitation, 119–122
    pumps and stimulators, 109

F

facet joint injections, 103
family and friends
    benefits, 205–206
    communicating with, 207–208
    help, asking for, 208
    interacting with, 205–210
    requirements, 206
    SMART goals, 210
    support system, 205
family responses, 58–60
    behaviors, 58–60
    emotions, 60
fear
    in emotional cycle, 55
    intercourse, 229–231
feet/ankle exercises, 154
fibroids, 48
fibromyalgia, 37
financial strain, 66
fingers/thumb exercises, 154
flexibility exercises, 153–154
friends. *See* family and friends
frontal cortex, 24

G

glucosamine, 128
goals. *See* SMART goals
guided imagery, 203
guilt, 56–57, 183

H

hamstring stretch, 155
hands-on therapies, 129–133

hands-on therapies continued
    aromatherapy, 129
    chiropractic, 130–131
    massage, 131–132
    movement therapies, 132
    prolotherapy, 132–133
    Rolfing, 133
headaches, 37–40
    migraine, 38–40
    tension-type, 38
    See also chronic pain
health, on Internet, 46–47
healthy weight, 216–218
heel cord stretch, 155
herbs/supplements
    devil's claw, 126–128
    evaluating, 127
    glucosamine and chondroitin, 128
    SAM-e, 128
hip exercises, 154
hip flexor stretch, 156
hope, 55, 58
hyaluronic acid, 99
hypnosis, 136–137

I

ibuprofen, 77
inactivity, 62
inflammation, 94
injections
    benefits, 96
    bursa, 100–101
    celiac plexus block, 104
    discogram, 104
    drug type, 96
    epidural, 102
    facet joint, 103
    intercostal, 97
    occipital, 97–98
    in pain treatment plan, 96
    peripheral joint and nerve, 96–100
    piriformis muscle, 104
    radiofrequency ablation, 105
    sacroiliac joint, 104
    selective nerve root, 103
    soft tissue, 100–101
    spinal, 101–105
    sympathetic block, 104
    therapy, 95–105
    transforaminal epidural, 102
    trigger point, 100
    types, 96
    use decision, 96
insurance coverage, 110
integrative medicine, 124

Internet health information, 46–47
interstitial cystitis, 48
intrathecal drug delivery systems, 108
irrational thinking
    examples, 184–185
    overcoming, 186
    types of, 186
irritable bowel syndrome (IBS), 40–41

J

jaw exercises, 153
journals
    mood, 149
    pain level and activities, 147–149
    sample, 148
    sleep, 149
    using, 146

K

ketamine-amitriptyline cream, 84–85
kneeling, 178–179

L

leg exercises, 160–161
lidocaine patches, 84
lifestyle
    alcohol limits, 223–224
    diet, 221–223
    sexuality, 228–231
    sleep, 211–215
    SMART goals, 232
    smoking cessation, 224–228
    spirituality, 231
    weight, 216–220
lifting, 179
limbic system, 24
local anesthetics, 84, 98–99
    in peripheral joint and nerve injections, 98–99
    in soft tissue injections, 101
long-handled tool use, 179
loss, admitting, 182–183
low back stretch, 156

M

magnet therapy, 135
management
    evolution, 21
    pain, 17–18, 233–238
    stress, 197–204
    time, 169–172
massage, 131–132
medication pumps, 108–110

defined, 108
elements, 108
expectations, 109
maintenance/troubleshooting, 110
running out of medication, 110
treatment elements, 109–110
medications, 71–94
    allergies, 73
    analgesics, 84–85
    anesthetics, 84
    anti-inflammatory, 94
    anti-seizure, 88–90
    anxiety, 90–92, 188
    beginning, 74
    benefits vs. risks, 94
    buying online, 91
    communicating about, 76
    counterirritant products, 85
    depression, 90–92
    dosage, 74
    efficacy, 72
    factors in prescribing, 72–74
    how to take, 75
    interactions, 72–73
    muscle relaxants, 93–94
    name of, 74
    as one treatment plan option, 74
    opioids, 79–84
    pain emotional symptoms, 90–93
    pain rehabilitation programs and, 120
    in peripheral joint and nerve injections, 98–100
    physical conditions, 93–94
    placebo effects, 73–74
    practical issues, 74
    purpose, 75
    rehabilitation and, 72
    results, 75
    role in chronic pain treatment, 72
    safety, 72
    serotonin and norepinephrine reuptake
            inhibitors (SNRIs), 88
    simple pain relievers, 76–79
    sleep, 92–93, 215
    in sleep loss, 62
    smoking cessation, 226–227
    soft tissue injections, 101
    topical, 84–85
    tramadol, 86
    tricyclic antidepressants, 86–88
    types, 72
    wise use of, 74–76
meditation, 137–138
migraines
    causes, 38–40
    diet, 39
    hormone fluctuations, 39

illustrated, 39
    lifestyle, 39–40
    medications triggering, 40
    pain, 38
    See also headaches
mind-body therapies, 135–140
    biofeedback, 136
    defined, 135–136
    hypnosis, 136–137
    meditation, 137–138
    music therapy, 138
    tai chi, 138–140
    yoga, 140
    See also complementary and alternative
            medicine
moderation, 173–174
motor nerves, 20
mouth, jaw and face pain, 41–43
    burning mouth syndrome, 41
    causes, 42–43
    temporomandibular disorders, 42
    trigeminal neuralgia, 41–42
movement therapies, 132
muscle relaxants, 93–94
muscle spasms, 34, 93–94
music therapy, 138

N

naproxen sodium, 77
naps, 214, 215
narcotics. See opioids
neck exercises, 153
neck pain, 43
nerves
    autonomic, 20
    motor, 20
    nociceptors, 22
    peripheral, 21–23
    sensory, 20
nerve stimulators, 105–107
    expectations, 109
    illustrated, 107
    maintenance/troubleshooting, 110
    spinal cord and peripheral nerve, 106
    TENS, 105–106
    treatment elements, 109–110
nervous system, 20, 83
neurologists, 112
nicotine medications, 226–227
nociceptors, 22
nonbenzodiazepines, 93
non-rapid eye movement (NREM) sleep, 212
nonsteroidal anti-inflammatory drugs
            (NSAIDs), 77
nurses, 115

O

online medication purchase, 91
opioids, 79–84
    additional risk, 82
    as agonists, 81
    defined, 79, 81
    effects, 83
    forms, 81
    nervous system changes, 83
    in pain treatment plan, 83–84
    rebound pain, 83
    side effects, 81
    types, 81
    use, 79
    use debate, 81–83
organization, life, 173
orofacial pain, 42
osteoarthritis, 32–33
ovarian remnant syndrome, 48
overachiever's curse, 56
overuse strain injuries, 44–45

P

pain
    acute, 27–28, 34
    back, 34–36
    behaviors, 54
    communicating, 54, 208
    defined, 19
    depression and, 183
    enhancers, natural, 25
    feeling of, 21–24
    as fifth vital sign, 21
    individual response to, 25–27
    memories, 26
    messages, brain and, 23–24
    messages, spinal cord and, 23
    mouth, jaw and face, 41–43
    neck, 43
    pathway, 22, 25
    pelvic, 45–48
    persistence, 20
    rebound, 83
    severe sensations, 23
    usefulness, 19
    See also chronic pain
pain clinics, 113–114
    cost, 116
    defined, 113
    evaluation factors, 115–116
    focus, 113–114
    success rate, 116
    See also pain specialists
pain control program, 143–150

pain costs
    damaged relationships, 66–67
    depression, 64–65
    emotional upheaval, 63–64
    financial strain, 66
    overcoming, 68
    physical deconditioning, 62
    sleep loss, 62–63
    substance misuse, 67
    work difficulties, 65–66
painkillers, natural, 25
pain management focus
    bad days and, 234–235
    challenges, 238
    contract, 235
    day planning, 236
    goal maintenance, 235
    help from others, 237
    maintaining, 233–238
    monitoring progress, 235
    positive orientation, 236
    rewards, 238
    support groups, 236–237
pain rehabilitation programs, 117–122
    commitment to, 118
    defined, 117–118
    effectiveness, 120–121
    expectations, 119–122
    finding, 122
    goals, 119
    location, 118–119
    pain specialists, 118
    readiness evaluation, 118
pain specialists, 111–116
    defined, 112
    in pain rehabilitation programs, 118
    as part of team, 114–115
    types of, 112
    See also pain clinics
pain-stress cycle, 197
passive behavior, 191
pelvic congestion syndrome, 48
pelvic floor tension myalgia, 45
pelvic inflammatory disease (PID), 45–48
pelvic pain, 45–48
    causes, 45–48
    statistics, 45
    See also chronic pain
peripheral joint and nerve injections, 96–100
    in diagnosis, 97
    function illustration, 97, 98
    intercostal, 97
    joints, 96–97
    local anesthetic, 98–99
    medications, 98–100
    occipital, 97–98

steroid, 99–100
targeted nerves, 97–98
See also injections
peripheral nerves, 21–23
injections, 98
stimulators, 106
peripheral neuropathy, 48–49
physiatrists, 112
physical activity, 62
physical deconditioning, 62
physical/occupational therapists, 115, 157
piriformis muscle injections, 104
positive orientation, 236–237, 238
positive self-talk, 184–185
postherpetic neuralgia, 49
posture, 162
pramoxine, 84
progress, monitoring, 235
progressive muscle relaxation, 203
prolotherapy, 132–133
psychiatrists, 112
psychologists, 115
pulling, 178
pushing, 178

Q

quadriceps stretch, 155–156

R

radiofrequency ablation, 105
range-of-motion exercise, 153
rapid eye movement (REM) sleep, 212
reaching, 177–178
rebound pain, 83
reflex sympathetic dystrophy (RSD), 36
rehabilitation, 72
relationships
damaged, 66–67
family and friends, 205–210
requirements, 206
social network, 207
relaxation
activities promoting, 213
benefits, 202
techniques, 202–203
See also stress management
rewards, 238
rheumatoid arthritis, 33–34
areas affected by, 33–34
defined, 33
development, 34
illustrated, 33
Rolfing, 133

S

sacroiliac joint injections, 104
SAM-e, 128
sciatica, 35
sedatives, 93
selective nerve root injections, 103
selective serotonin reuptake inhibitors (SSRIs),
90–92
self-care. See lifestyle
self-esteem
benefits, 194
defined, 193
suggestions, 193–194
sensitization, 29–30
sensory nerves, 20
serotonin and norepinephrine reuptake
inhibitors (SNRIs), 88
sexuality, 228–231
chronic pain and, 228
creative lovemaking, 230
expressing, 228–231
fears, 229–231
intimacy, increasing, 229
patience and understanding, 231
shingles, 49
shoulder exercises, 153
simple pain relievers, 76–79
acetaminophen, 76
COX-2 inhibitors, 77–79
defined, 76
nonsteroidal anti-inflammatory drugs
(NSAIDs), 77, 78
See also medications
sleep
benefits, 211–212
diet and, 214
interference factors, 212
journal entries, 149
loss, 62–63
medications, 92–93, 215
naps, 214, 215
regular hours, 213
stages, 212
strategies, 212–215
in stress reduction, 200
SMART goals
attainable, 144
daily living, 180
defined, 144
examples, 145
exercise, 164
friendships and communication, 210
lifestyle, 232
measurable, 144
realistic, 145

SMART goals continued
    setting, 146
    specific, 144
    stress reduction, 204
    timely, 145–146
smoking, quitting, 224–228
    medications, 226–227
    steps, 224–228
social network, 207
soft tissue injections, 100–101
somatosensory cortex, 24
spinal injections, 101–105
    celiac plexus block, 104
    discogram, 104
    epidural, 102
    facet joint, 103
    intrathecal, 101
    piriformis muscle, 104
    radiofrequency ablation, 105
    sacroiliac joint, 104
    selective nerve root, 103
    sympathetic block, 104
    transforaminal epidural, 102
    See also injections
spirituality, 231
steroids, 99–100
    in peripheral joint and nerve injections, 99–100
    in soft tissue injections, 101
strengthening exercises, 158–162
    abdominal, 159–160
    back, 160
    chest and arm, 161
    leg, 160–161
    weightlifting, 158
stress
    effects, 198
    internal/external factors, 199
    negative, 198
    positive, 198
    triggers, 198–199
stress management, 197–204
    attitude, 202
    breathing, 201
    lifestyle changes, 200–202
    relaxation, 202–203
    SMART goals, 204
stretching exercises, 154–156
    hamstring, 155
    heel cord, 155
    hip flexor, 156
    low back, 156
    quadriceps, 155–156
substance misuse, 67
support groups, 236–237
sympathetic block injections, 104

T

tai chi, 138–140
    benefits, 140
    defined, 138
    in general health improvement, 138–140
    illustrated, 139
    See also mind-body therapies
temporomandibular disorders, 42
TENS, 105–106
tension-type headaches, 38
time management, 169–172
    daily planner for, 171–172
    strategies, 169–170
topical medications, 84–85
tramadol, 86
transforaminal epidural injections, 102
tricyclic antidepressants, 86–88
    defined, 86
    medications, 86
    side effects, 86–88
    See also medications
trigeminal neuralgia, 41–42
trigger point injections, 100
trolamine salicylate, 85
trunk exercises, 154

W

warning signs, 234–235
weight
    BMI and, 216, 217, 218
    controlling, 216–220
    healthy, 216–218
    personal/family history and, 218
    waist circumference and, 216–217
weightlifting, 158
weight loss
    commitment, 219
    goals, 219–220
    healthy, 220
    as lifelong process, 220
    successful, 218–220
work difficulties, 65–66
worry time, 215
wrist exercises, 154
writing, journal, 147–149

Y

yoga, 140

Z

ziconotide, 108